Keto Baking and Dessert Recipes for Dummies

Master All the Best Tricks for Low-Carb Baking Success: Bread, Pies, and Waffles

Introduction

You might think the ketogenic diet means saying goodbye to carbs and sugars, but thanks to the incredible recipes in this book, you can enjoy natural and delicious baked goods that will satisfy your sweet tooth and relieve your carb cravings.

Switching to keto is easier than ever without giving up your favorite sweets!

It's no secret that the keto diet helps us cope with debilitating diseases such as heart disease, high blood sugar, and distorted cholesterol. This is of great importance for our well-being and improving the quality of life.

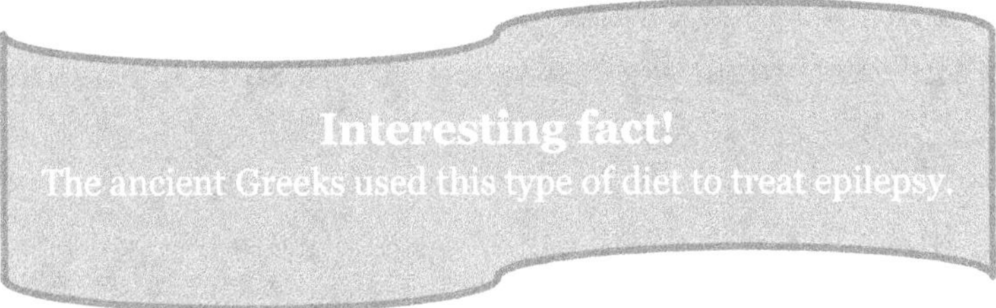

In this book, you will find delicious and healthy recipes to help your diet work effectively. They are so quick and easy to prepare that you won't be spending all your precious time in the kitchen. Each recipe lists the ingredients, instructions, cooking times, servings, and nutritional values.

Benefits of the Keto Diet

Helps suppress hunger

The keto diet naturally suppresses hunger. This is extremely important when you are on a weight-loss diet. Weight loss occurs gradually, not suddenly. This is because a sequence of reactions, called ketosis, occurs in the human body, and this reaction prevents weight gain. Ketones, a category that ketogenic foods belong to, are more effective food sources. They have also been linked to improved brain function. When the human body is in a state of ketosis, it switches its energy sources to ketones, which help generate energy.

Increases energy levels

Thanks to the ketogenic diet, the increased energy levels in the body are maintained for a longer period of time. Chronic fatigue is a thing of the past, regardless of whether it results from illness or overwork.

Increases the level of "healthy fats" in the body

Thanks to the keto diet, the level of good lipids (HDL) increases, and bad lipids (LDL) decreases.

Reduces insulin levels and blood sugar

The keto diet can be especially beneficial for people with diabetes. Studies have shown that cutting back on carbohydrates in the diet drastically lowers glucose and insulin levels. Some people with diabetes may soon cut their insulin in half by switching to a low-carb diet.

High blood pressure, or hypertension, is a major contributor to disease, including stroke, kidney failure, and heart disease. Eating foods that are low in carbohydrates is a great way to lower blood pressure, which in turn can help reduce the risk of these diseases.

Main Ingredients

Almond flour is quite popular in the keto diet as the main substitute for the traditional wheat flours. It has a much higher fat content than wheat flour, which tends to burn recipes much quicker. You will find that many of the oven temperatures in these recipes are lower than the traditional recipes for that very reason.

Coconut flour has extremely high levels of saturated fats (which are healthy for you!), and these fats actually aid in metabolism and assist in balancing out the blood sugar levels naturally. Coconut flour has many other benefits such as being low in sugar and carbs, high in fiber, and is absolutely packed with vitamins and minerals.

Sesame flour is very dry and powdery. It is low in carbohydrates when compared to other flour alternatives. Flour also has a strong sesame flavor, which can be good or bad depending on your preference. In keto baked goods, this flour is best used in combination with other types of flour.

Lupine flour is becoming more popular in keto baked goods and is made from lupine beans, which are associated with peanuts and soybeans. It is low in carbs (12 grams per cup), but about 90 percent of that is fiber. Lupine flour also has a distinct flavor that needs getting used to.

Flour from pumpkin seeds is a good nut-free alternative. It has a slightly bitter taste when used alone, so you need to increase the amount of sweetener. Pumpkin seed flour is also slightly greenish and is not suitable for many recipes, but is a great substitute for cocoa-based recipes.

Peanut flour is a very tasty and healthy flour that can be prepared in different ways. It can be just ground peanuts, in which case they are light and rather large, or roasted peanuts, in which case the flour will be darker in color, very fine, and powdery. Because peanut flour is more absorbent than almond flour, you may need a lot of liquid to dilute it. It is best used in combination with other keto flours.

Sunflower seed flour is one of the best nut-free alternatives to almond flour. It has the same texture and consistency, which allows you to easily replace it in recipes to be nut-free. When combined with baking powder or baking soda, sunflower seed flour chemically reacts, and baked goods take on an odd greenish tint. Add a tablespoon of acid, such as lemon juice or apple cider vinegar, to neutralize this reaction. Recipes with the addition of chocolate or cocoa powder are also great for masking green.

Monk fruit sweetener is also a popular choice; you must know that this sweetener will make your dishes sweeter versus the other choices of sweeteners. However, people who do prefer monk fruit sweetener find that other sweeteners have a cooling effect and bad aftertaste. If you find this to be true, this will be the choice of sweeteners for you.

Natvia icing mix is a combination of stevia and erythritol sweeteners, resulting in the perfect icing that you are used to in old-fashioned recipes. But it is even better! It does not contain any artificial flavors or colors and does not cause plaque buildup on your teeth. Alternatively, you can use Swerve Icing Sugar Style in the recipes if you prefer the taste.

Sukrin Gold brown sugar substitute is also used by monk fruit lovers, as it packs the same sweet taste. This can be used as a substitute for your keto baking needs, as it does not burn as hot as the other sweeteners and still has only eight calories per 100 grams.

Stevia liquid drops can be used in many sweets and can be substituted particularly for the confectioner sweetener. It also contains no calories or carbs and does not alter your blood sugar levels. With over a dozen flavors to choose from, it can be the next must-have section in your pantry.

Swerve has the same amount of sweetness compared to traditional white sugars found in recipes. It measures out to be the same if converting recipes after you get deeper into the world of keto, as you will find yourself going through your grandmother's recipes to convert them. There are also no calories in this sweetener, so it can prevent you from feeling guilty when you are eating those keto cookies!

Truvia is the brand name for the natural sweetener of the stevia plant. Most people who are into eating healthy have heard of stevia, or the common name of erythritol. This is a sugar alcohol that is found in melons and grapes and also has no calories.

Eggs play a very important role in baking. They provide structure as well as moisture and fat content and help the baked goods rise. To properly beat the egg whites, a dry whisk and bowl must be used. Even one drop of yolk, oil, or water can interfere with a good whipping. It will be possible to correctly separate the whites from the yolks while the eggs are cold while whipping the whites is better at room temperature. Plan ahead.

Chocolate

There are many different types of chocolate, and it is very important to use the right chocolate in your recipes. This is critical to both the flavor and texture of your dessert. An exception is chocolate decoration.

Cocoa powder is a solid, ground into powder. It is made from roasted cocoa beans, so it has a very rich chocolate flavor.

Unsweetened chocolate, mostly used in baked goods, is made from cocoa solids and cocoa butter, without sweeteners, dairy products, or other additives. It is bitter enough to be consumed just like that but gives a rich chocolate flavor to desserts and baked goods.

Sugar-free chocolate should not be confused with unsweetened chocolate. Sugar-free chocolate contains sweeteners. Usually, it also contains additives that give it a creamy taste and smoothness. It comes in different varieties, from very dark to milky, and depending on this, it contains a different percentage of cocoa. Sugar-free chocolate is good for keto baked goods, but replacing it with unsweetened chocolate is not recommended as varying amounts can affect the texture of your baked goods, and the sweetener can change the flavor.

Almond oil in its purest form is simply ground roasted or raw almonds. It is a much healthier alternative to regular butter, as there are no additives like sugar and it has three grams of net carbohydrates per serving.

Cashew oil butter is a substitute for traditional butters that gives your dishes a naturally sweet flavor. It also helps your sweet treats to have a more rich and creamy dough. You may choose between 100% cashew butter, or some varieties have sunflower oil included. Note that the butter with sunflower oil will add a more oily consistency to your sweet recipes, and they will be denser.

Coconut oil can be used as a substitute in these recipes instead of butter. This is a good choice for people who have lactose intolerance or a dairy allergy.

Grass-fed oil has been shown to have higher contents of nutrients such as linoleic acid (CLA) and is loaded with beneficial fats and vitamins versus traditional butter, which generally comes from GMO-fed cows.

Hazelnut butter oil is another healthy alternative to regular butter, as it is high in vitamin E and manganese. You will find the more you research the keto diet that manganese is essential in aiding in fat and carb metabolism.

The importance of dairy products in baking is very high, and the fats in dairy products give the baked goods tenderness and moisture. It is not uncommon for dairy products to be the main source of fat throughout a recipe. Also, you should not panic if you do not eat dairy products. There are many alternatives now.

Heavy cream is a great ingredient in many recipes. Heavy whipping cream (36–40 percent) differs from whipped cream (30–36 percent) only in a higher milk fat content. A dairy-free alternative is full-fat coconut milk, or better yet, coconut cream. However, because coconut cream is almost solid at room temperature, it may need to be warmed up a little if it is to be added in liquid form.

Cream cheese is very popular in the keto diet. It is great for curd desserts and frostings, and it also helps gum up baked goods and gives them a wonderful texture and flavor. Previously, all dairy-free cheeses were soy-based, but now that has changed. One example is cheese from kite hill, which is based on almond milk and works just as well as cream cheese. It does not change taste or texture.

Sour cream is the same cream that is fermented by certain bacteria. Fatty sour cream gives special tenderness to baked goods. Fatty Greek yogurt can be used instead.

Almond and nut milk. Unsweetened almond milk is preferred in baked goods. This will help add moisture without excess carbohydrates. For example, a cup of cow's milk contains 12 grams of carbohydrates, and a cup of almond only two grams. Of course, you can replace the almond milk half with heavy cream and half with water, as using only the cream will make the dough too thick.

If you don't eat nuts, you can substitute unsweetened hemp milk for almond milk.

If you've baked wheat flour all your life, you've enjoyed all the magical qualities of gluten. Although not very good for your health, gluten is a wonderful substance that has very valuable qualities. This is why we often cannot substitute a cup of wheat flour for a cup of almond or coconut flour.

Gluten is protein. It is composed of two protein molecules, glutenin and gliadin, which are naturally found in wheat and other grains such as barley and rye. These molecules are practically inactive in dry flour, but they begin to change dramatically as soon as they come into contact with liquid. Individual molecules stick together and form long strands. These threads then join together and form a net that is very strong and elastic. Gluten also absorbs and retains moisture, which prevents baked goods from drying out in the oven. With all this in mind, it is very difficult to find an alternative to gluten in keto baked goods. But there are ways and means that can replace the properties of gluten. Eggs can be a great glue in desserts. Adding dry protein powders such as whey or egg white can also help your desserts rise and stay in shape. If you add a small amount of gelatin to the cookie dough, you can achieve a chewy quality.

Tips Before Starting Work

1. Be sure to read the recipe to the end. Check for all ingredients. This will give you an idea of how long it will take and what steps to take.

2. Prepare all required ingredients. Recipes may require room-temperature ingredients, chopped, etc.

3. Measure the ingredients exactly and add them in the order shown. The final result of your dessert depends on this. For example, whipping butter with sweeteners before adding the eggs helps create air bubbles as your baked goods rise.

4. Be sure to scrub the beaters and bowls. Many ingredients, such as butter, stick to the bottom of the bowl while stirring.

5. Set the timer for the minimum baking time. All recipes show approximate baking times or time ranges. Check your dessert.

6. Preheat the oven. Baked goods often need a high temperature in the beginning to help them rise.

7. In recipes, always pay attention to the temperature of the ingredients: softened, room, chilled, cold, or melted. These instructions should not be ignored as they are critical to the outcome.

The Main Helpers in Your Kitchen

Required tools:

- whisk and spatulas
- measuring spoons, cups, and kitchen scales
- mixer (tabletop or portable)
- mixing mats, beaters, rubber spatulas, wooden spoons

The tools you'll only need for some of the recipes in this book:

- trays and pans
- cake molds
- molds for muffins
- bread maker

Baking materials:

- parchment
- Silpat non-stick baking mats

<u>Oven</u>

Get to know your oven better. No two ovens are exactly the same when it comes to temperature. The best solution is an accurate oven thermometer. It is installed in the center of the oven and displays the exact temperature. The hotspots of your oven should also be considered. If your pastry browns more on one side, turn the baking sheet halfway so that the treat is baked evenly.

Convection ovens: Because convection ovens use fans to circulate the air, baking is faster and more even. Lower the oven temperature by 25°F and start checking baked goods 5–10 minutes earlier.

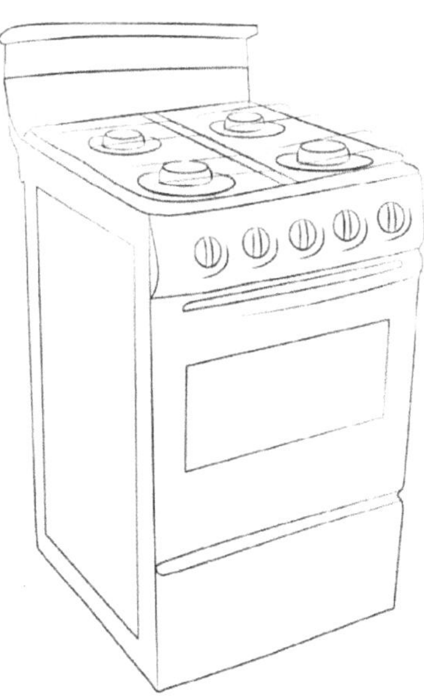

Bread Maker

Bread makers are undeniably convenient. The bread is very tasty and perfectly formed. The bread maker can make an incredible variety of bread that you can make without spending hours in the kitchen. There are several reasons your bread maker will quickly become your favorite kitchen appliance:

- Saves energy. The energy consumption of a standard bread maker is about the same or less than that of a coffee maker; about nine-kilowatt hours for 15 hours a month.
- Saves time.
- Control over ingredients. You know exactly what is in food.

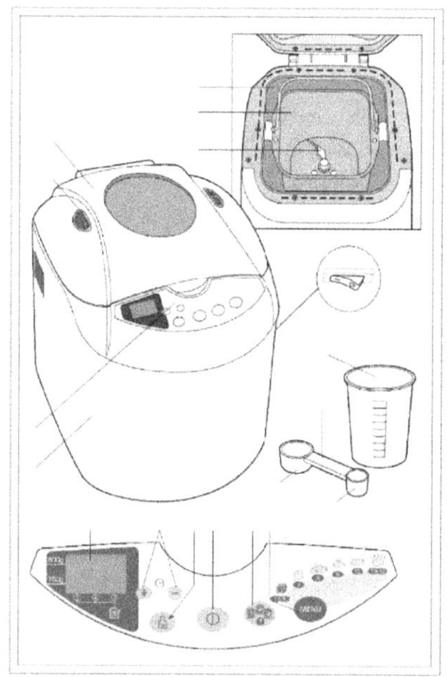

Waffle Maker

How to choose a keto waffle iron. The waffle maker is a kitchen device for making waffles. It consists of two plates with heating elements connected by hinges. Outside, the slabs are covered with lids. This design allows the product to be fried on both sides. Cooking time is 3–5 minutes on average. The waffle iron's speed directly depends on its power, which ranges from 450 to 1,600 watts. For home use, 700–800 watts is quite suitable.

- ✓ When buying a waffle iron, be sure to check the quality of the non-stick coating. The right choice is an even coating without bubbles, chips, and other defects.
- ✓ The lids of the waffle iron should be tightly-closed so that the dough does not overflow.
- ✓ After baking is complete, let the hot surfaces cool down and then wipe them off with a damp cloth. Avoid getting water inside the waffle iron. Dry the device before storing it.

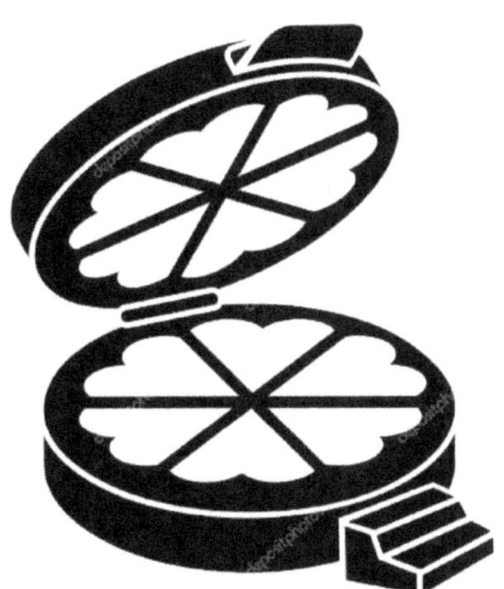

Pies and Cakes

We all love birthday cake or pie as an afternoon treat. You should not deny yourself this. Keto desserts made with low-carb flour will not cause high and low levels of glucose and insulin. Carbohydrates easily enter the body and are easily absorbed. If a person is switching from a diet rich in desserts, it will be very difficult for him to adhere to the new meal plan. Keto desserts are great because they satisfy sugar cravings without causing a spike in blood sugar and insulin levels.

Storage. The best place to store cakes and pies is undoubtedly the refrigerator, where your dessert can be stored for up to five days at a temperature of plus 2–6. To prevent the cake or pie from absorbing foreign odors in the refrigerator, it is better to cover it with cling film or a cardboard box. Allow your dessert to cool completely beforehand. Pies can be stored in the freezer for 2–3 months. After the cake is thawed at room temperature, you can reheat it in the microwave or oven at a low temperature.

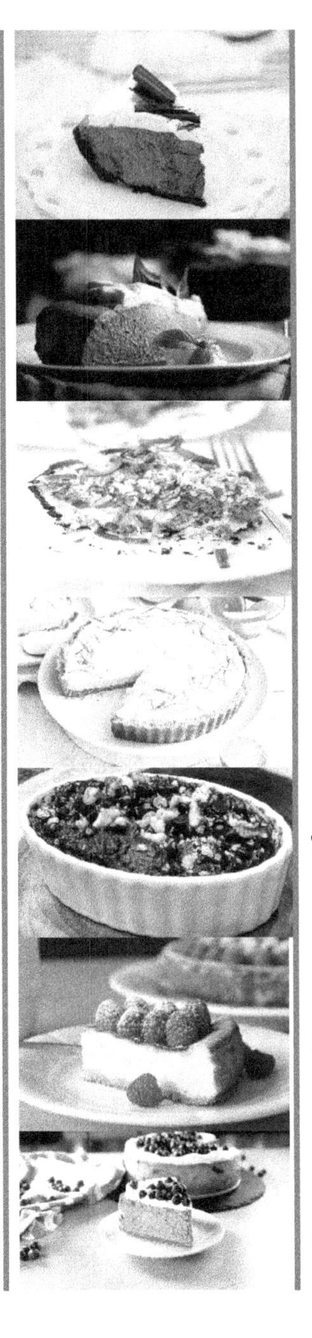

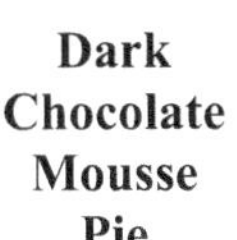

French
Silk Pie

Dark
Chocolate
Mousse
Pie

Chocolate
Coconut
Mounds
Pie

Coconut
Key Lime
Pie

Brownie
Truffle Pie

Sweet
Ricotta
Cheese Pie

No-Bake
Blueberry
Cheesecak
e Pie

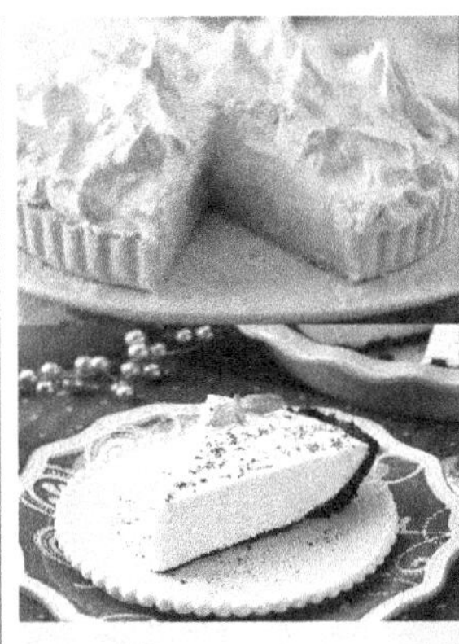

Lemon
Meringue
Pie

Grasshoppe
r Mint Pie

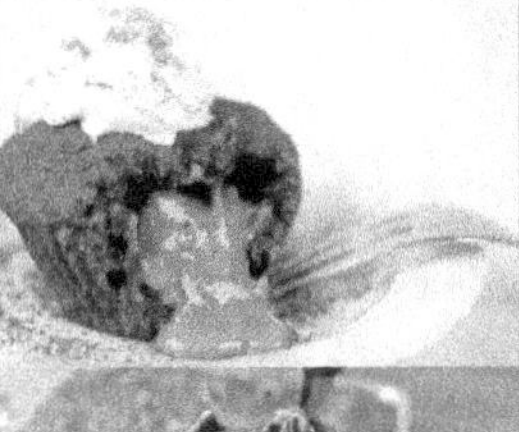

Peanut
Butter
Molten
Lava Cake

Texas Sheet
Cake

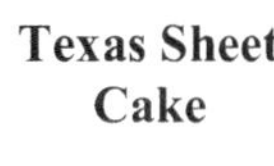

Pecan Pie
Cheesecake

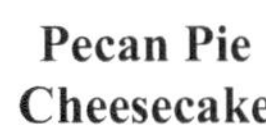

Chocolate
Walnut
Torte

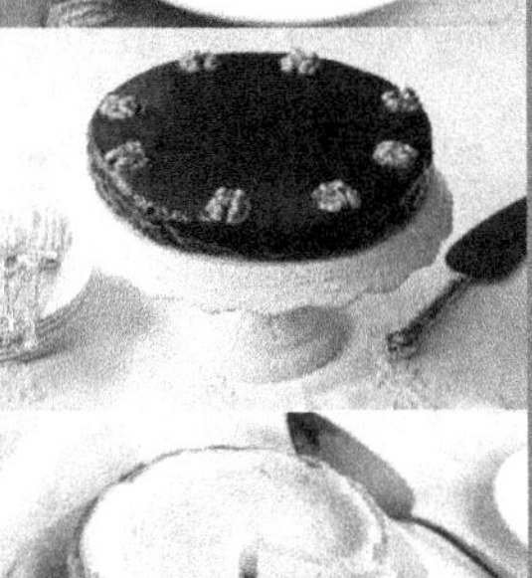

Classic New
York Keto
Cheesecake

French Silk Pie

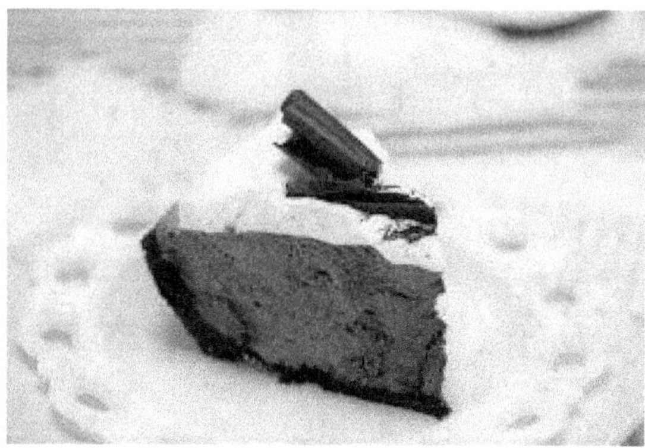

Ingredients	**Calories: 337** **Fat: 34 g** **Carbohydrates: 8 g** **Protein: 6 g**	**Cook Time: 10 minutes** **Servings: 10**

Flaky Pie Crust (or your favorite crust)

- 1 ½ cup almond flour
- 5 TBSP butter
- 3 TBSP oat fiber
- 1 large egg white
- 1 tsp water
- ¼ tsp salt

Topping

- ¾ cup heavy cream
- Chocolate shavings (optional). I used 2 squares of chocolate at 86% cacao
- 2 TBSP sukrin melis (icing sugar) (or Swerve)

French Silk Pie Filling

- 6 oz (1 ½ sticks) salted butter, very soft
- 1 ¼ cups Sukrin Melis (icing sugar) (or Swerve Confectioners)
- ¼ cup heavy cream
- 4 oz unsweetened baking chocolate squares, melted
- 4 large pasteurized eggs, cold
- 2 tsp vanilla extract
- ½ tsp stevia glycerite (or more Sukrin or Swerve to taste)

Crust

1. Preheat oven to 350°F. Spray a pie plate with baking spray. I use a 9-inch pyrex baking dish. (I sprinkle sesame seeds on the bottom of the pie plate so the crust doesn't stick to the bottom.)

2. Measure the almond flour, oat fiber, and salt into the bowl of a food processor. Pulse to combine. Cut the butter into chunks and pulse with the dry ingredients until the butter is the size of small peas. Mix the egg white with the 1 teaspoon of water and pour onto the dry ingredients. Process until the dough just comes together. Refrigerate the dough for 30 minutes or up to five days.

3. Roll the pastry between two sheets of plastic wrap until it is the right size for your pie plate. Remove the top piece of plastic and invert the dough over the pie plate. Gently coax the dough into the bottom and the sides of the plate. Remove the plastic and shape the edge. Dock the dough with a fork.

4. Bake the crust for 10–15 minutes, until it begins to turn a nice golden-brown. Let cool completely, then cover with plastic wrap until ready to use.

Filling

1. Finely chop the unsweetened baking chocolate and put in a microwaveable bowl. Heat on high 30 seconds at a time until almost melted. The residual heat from the bowl should take care of melting the rest.

2. Put the butter and Sukrin Melis or Swerve in a stand mixer or a large mixing bowl. Fit the paddle attachment onto the mixer and beat the butter and sweetener on medium speed for about two minutes. Scrape the bowl. Add the melted chocolate and mix for one minute. Scrape down the bowl thoroughly. Add ¼ cup of heavy cream, vanilla, and stevia glycerite, beating for two minutes more. Remove the paddle attachment, and scrape the filling back into the bowl.

3. Add the whisk attachment and turn the stand mixer back on medium speed. Add one egg at a time and let the mixer run for about three minutes between each addition, scraping the bowl after the third and forth additions.

4. Finish mixing with a quick burst at high speed and spread the filling into the pie shell and refrigerate. (NOTE: If the filling breaks [separates], refrigerate for 40 minutes and add ¼ teaspoon of xanthan gum. Whip at medium speed for a few seconds to loosen the filling and then at high for just a few seconds until it comes together. Another pinch of xanthan gum may be needed.)

5. Spoon the filling into the pie crust and smooth with a spoon or offset spatula. Refrigerate at least six hours or overnight, uncovered.

6. Whip the ¾ cup of heavy cream with your favorite sweetener and top the pie. Additionally, chocolate curls can be added by running a vegetable peeler down the length of a piece of chocolate.

Dark Chocolate Mousse Pie

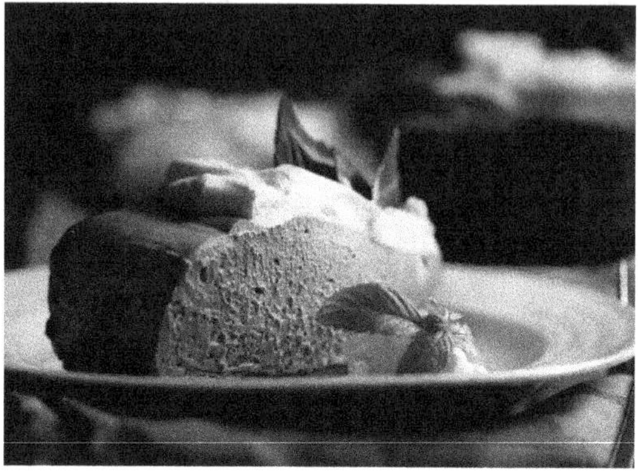

Ingredients

Calories: 325
Fat: 29 g
Carbohydrates: 9 g
Protein: 11 g

Cook Time: 20 minutes
Servings: 10

Peanut Flour Crust

- ½ cup natural peanut butter
- 2 TBSP butter
- 2 eggs, beaten
- ½ tsp vanilla extract
- 1 cup peanut flour
- ½ tsp baking powder
- ¼ tsp salt
- ¼ cup low-carb sugar substitute, more or less to taste

Hershey's Dark Chocolate Mousse

- 7–9 grams grass-fed gelatin, about 2 tsp or a bit more
- ¼ cup cold water
- 1/3 cup boiling water
- ½ cup low-carb sugar substitute, more or less to taste
- 2/3 cup Hershey's Dark Cocoa
- 2 cups cold whipping cream
- 2 tsp vanilla extract

Crust

1. Microwave peanut butter and butter in medium bowl until melted.
2. Beat butter into peanut butter until well combined.
3. Stir in vanilla, beaten eggs, and sweetener.
4. Add the rest of the ingredients and stir until dough forms.
5. Press dough into 9-inch pie pan. Bake at 325°F for 15–20 minutes.
6. Place on rack to cool.

Mousse Filling

1. Sprinkle gelatin over cold water in small bowl; let stand two minutes to soften.
2. Add boiling water; stir until gelatin is completely dissolved and mixture is clear.
3. Cool slightly.
4. Combine sweetener and cocoa in large bowl; add whipping cream and vanilla.
5. Beat on medium speed of mixer, scraping bottom of bowl occasionally, until mixture is stiff.
6. Pour in gelatin mixture; beat until well blended.
7. Spoon into pie crust. Refrigerate at least four hours before serving.

Chocolate Coconut Mounds Pie

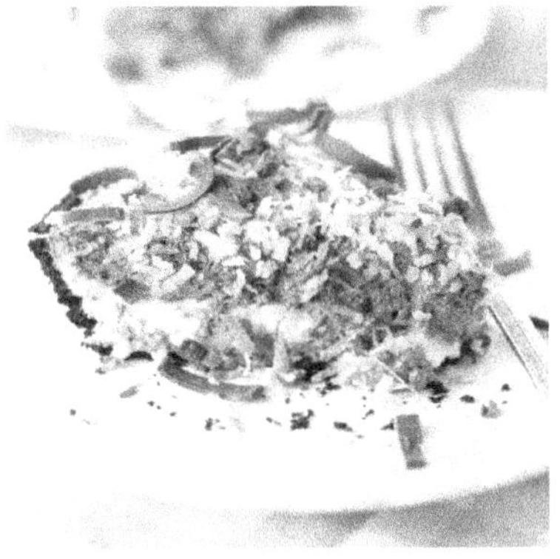

Ingredients	Calories: 325	Cook Time: 40 minutes
	Fat: 29 g	Servings: 8
	Carbohydrates: 9 g	
	Protein: 11 g	

Crust

- 2 cups unsweetened coconut milk
- 4 eggs
- 1 tsp vanilla extract
- 1 ½ tsp coconut stevia
- 2 cups unsweetened shredded coconut
- ½ cup unsweetened cocoa powder
- ¼ cup coconut flour
- ½ tsp salt

Coconut Cream Topping

- 1 can (15 oz) coconut milk (opened, overnight in fridge)
- Optional: 2 ounces Lily's sugar-free coconut chocolate bar

1. In a stand mixer with a whisk attachment blend the first four ingredients together.
2. Change to the paddle attachment and add the rest of the ingredients on low speed.
3. Pour mixture into a pie plate and bake for 40 minutes.
4. Allow to cool before adding coconut cream topping.
5. Keep refrigerated.

Coconut Key Lime Pie

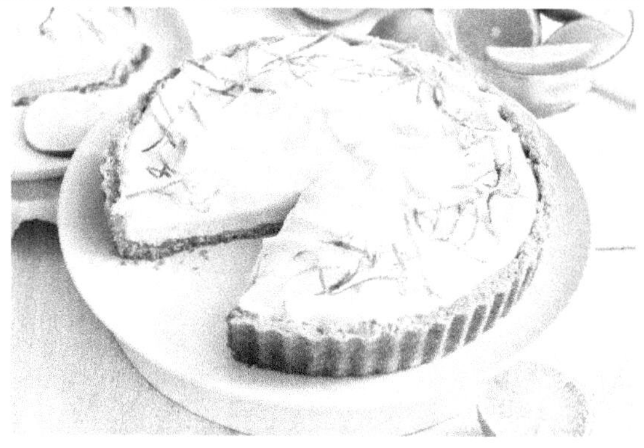

Calories: 460
Fat: 42 g
Carbohydrates: 6 g
Protein: 11 g

Cook Time:50 minutes
Servings: 9

Crust	Filling
• 2 cups raw hazelnuts • 1 egg • 4 TBSP chia seeds • 4 TBSP organic butter, melted • 1 TBSP coconut oil • 1 TBSP Swerve	• 1.5 cup coconut cream • 1.5 cup sour cream • 3 large eggs • 1 cup fresh key lime juice • 3 TBSP Swerve • 1 TBSP key lime zest • ½ cup unsweetened coconut shavings

1. Pre heat oven to 375°F.
2. In a food processor grind the hazelnuts until they turn in to a flour, then add the chia seeds, Swerve, egg, and melted butter. Mix everything together until a dough is formed.
3. Now grease a 6 by 9-inch pyrex with coconut oil.
4. Press the crust flat into the pyrex.
5. Bake for 20 minutes at 375°F.
6. In the meantime, prepare the filling.
7. In a large bowl mix all the filling ingredients and blend with an immersion blender until smooth and frothy.
8. Remove the crust from the oven once done.
9. Pour filling onto crust and put back in the oven at 350°F.
10. Bake for 45 minutes.
11. Remove from the oven, and let cool, then sprinkle evenly with the coconut flakes.

Brownie Truffle Pie

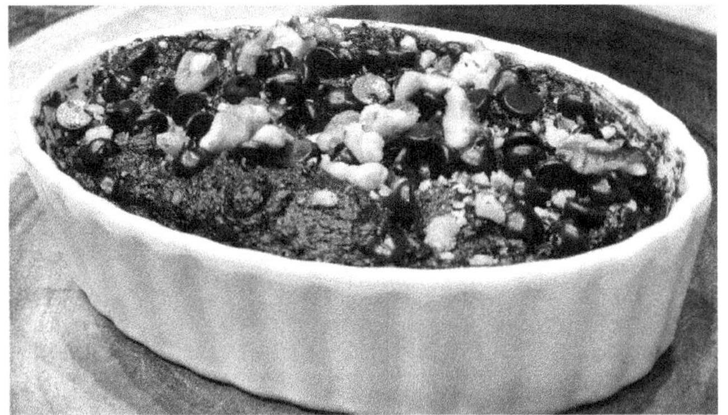

Ingredients	Calories: 370 Fat: 33 g Carbohydrates: 6 g Protein: 8 g	Cook Time: 30 minutes Servings: 4

Crust

- 1 ¼ cup almond flour
- 3 TBSP coconut flour
- 1 TBSP granulated Swerve Sweetener
- ¼ tsp salt
- 5 TBSP butter chilled and cut into small pieces
- 2–4 TBSP ice water

Filling

- ½ cup almond flour
- 6 TBSP cocoa powder
- 6 TBSP Swerve Sweetener
- 1 tsp baking powder
- 2 large eggs
- 5 TBSP water
- ¼ cup melted butter
- 1 TBSP Sukrin Fiber Syrup (optional, but helps create a more gooey center)
- ½ tsp vanilla extract
- 3 TBSP sugar-free chocolate chips

Topping

- 1 cup whipping cream
- 2 TBSP confectioner's Swerve Sweetener
- ¼ tsp vanilla extract
- ½ oz sugar-free dark chocolate

Crust

1. Preheat oven to 325°F and grease a glass or ceramic pie pan.
2. In a large bowl, combine almond flour, coconut flour, sweetener, and salt. Cut in butter using a pastry cutter or two sharp knives until mixture resembles coarse crumbs. Add two tablespoons water and mix until dough comes together. Add more water only if necessary to get dough to come together.
3. Press evenly into the bottom and up the sides of prepared pie pan, crimp edges, and prick bottom all over with a fork. Bake 12 minutes.

Filling

1. In a large bowl, whisk together the almond flour, cocoa powder, sweetener, and baking powder. Stir in eggs, water, melted butter, and vanilla extract until well combined. Stir in chocolate chips.
2. Pour batter into crust and bake 30 minutes, covering with foil about halfway through. Remove and let cool 10 minutes, then refrigerate half an hour until cool.

Topping

1. Combine cream, sweetener, and vanilla extract in a large bowl. Beat until cream holds stiff peaks. Spread over cooled filling.
2. Shave dark chocolate over top. Chill another hour or two until completely set.

Sweet Ricotta Cheese Pie

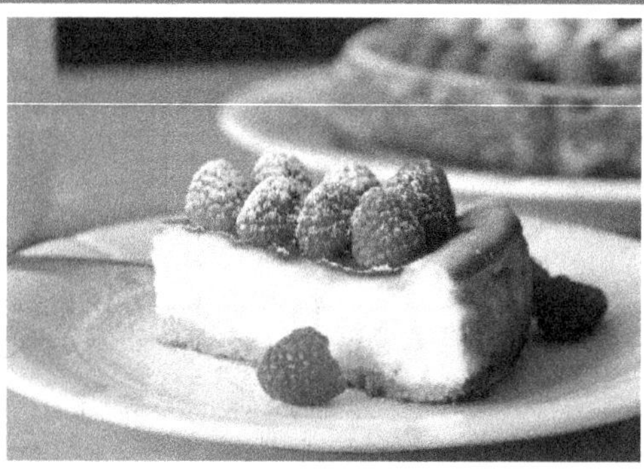

Ingredients	Calories: 170	Cook Time: 50 minutes
	Fat: 12 g	Servings: 8
	Carbohydrates: 4 g	
	Protein: 10 g	

- 1 ½ cups almond flour, sifted
- 3 TBSP low-carb sugar substitute (I used Swerve)
- ¼ tsp salt
- ¼ cup butter, melted
- 1 egg
- 1 tsp vanilla extract

- 4 eggs, beaten
- 1 tsp vanilla extract
- 15 oz ricotta cheese
- 1 TBSP coconut flour
- ¾ cup Swerve (add more if desired; up to 1 cup)
- 2 TBSP low-carb sugar substitute or 24 drops liquid stevia to help round out sweetness

1. In deep dish pie plate, mix together almond flour, 3 tablespoons equivalent sugar substitute and ¼ teaspoon salt.
2. Pour in butter, 1 egg, and 1 teaspoon vanilla.
3. Mix until dough forms.
4. Press into pie plate. Bake at 350°F for 10 minutes.
5. Set on rack to cool slightly.
6. In a large bowl mix 4 beaten eggs, 1 teaspoon vanilla, ricotta cheese, coconut flour, 1 cup equivalent sugar substitute, and 2 tablespoons other sweetener.
7. Beat until smooth.
8. Pour into crust and bake at 350°F for 45 minutes or until lightly browned and firm.

No-Bake Blueberry Cheesecake Pie

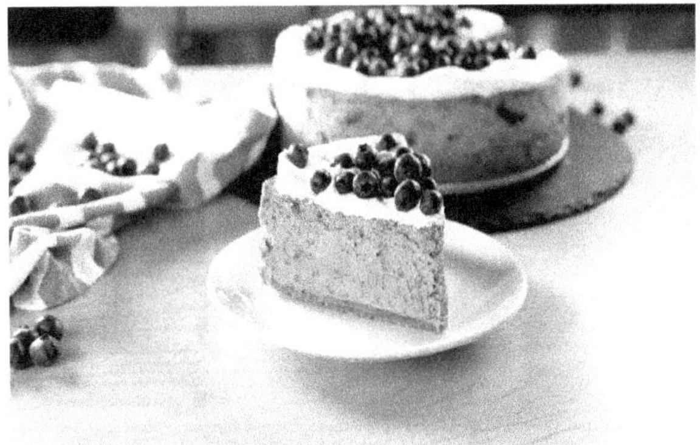

Calories: 325
Fat: 28 g
Carbohydrates: 7 g
Protein: 6 g

Prep Time: 40 minutes
Servings: 10

Crust
- 1 ½ cups almond flour
- ¼ cup powdered Swerve Sweetener
- ¼ cup butter, melted

Topping
Blueberry syrup (no sugar)
Pour over the cheesecake before serving.

Filling
- 12 oz cream cheese, softened
- 2 TBSP sour cream or Greek yogurt, room temperature
- 2 TBSP freshly-squeezed lemon juice
- 1 tsp lemon zest
- ¾ cup powdered Swerve Sweetener
- ½ cup plus 2 TBSP heavy whipping cream, divided
- 1 TBSP grassfed gelatin or 1 envelope Knox gelatin

Crust

1. In a medium bowl, whisk together almond flour and powdered Sweetener. Stir in butter until well combined and clumps form.
2. Press firmly into the bottom and up the sides of a 9-inch pie pan. Refrigerate until needed.

Filling

3. In a large bowl, beat cream cheese, sour cream or yogurt, lemon juice, and lemon zest together until smooth. Beat in sweetener until well combined.
4. In a small bowl, whisk together 2 TBSP heavy cream and the gelatin. Gently warm the mixture in the microwave for about 20 to 30 seconds, and then stir until the gelatin dissolves (you can also do this in a small saucepan; do not let the cream come to a simmer). Stir into cream cheese mixture until combined.
5. In another large bowl, beat cream until it holds stiff peaks. Gently fold whipped cream into cream cheese mixture until well combined.
6. Spread filling in prepared crust, cover with plastic and refrigerate two to three hours, until set.

Lemon Meringue Pie

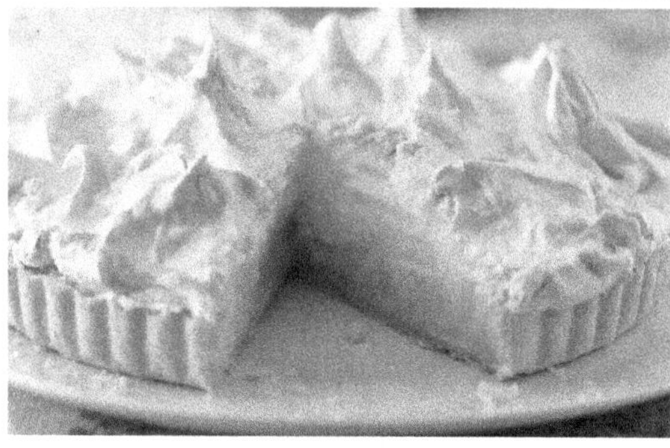

<table>
<tr><td>Ingredients</td><td>Calories: 218
Fat: 17 g
Carbohydrates: 7 g
Protein: 6 g</td><td>Cook
minutes
Servings: 1</td><td>Time:50</td></tr>
</table>

Pastry Crust

- 1 ¼ cup almond flour
- 2 TBSP coconut flour
- 2 TBSP arrowroot starch OR 2 TBSP oat fiber for THM
- 1 TBSP granulated Swerve Sweetener
- 1 tsp xanthan gum
- ¼ tsp salt
- 5 TBSP butter, chilled and cut into small pieces
- 2–4 TBSP ice water

Meringue Topping

- 4 large egg whites at room temperature
- ¼ tsp cream of tartar
- Pinch of salt
- ¼ cup powdered Swerve Sweetener
- ¼ cup granulated Swerve Sweetener
- ½ tsp vanilla extract

Filling

- 1 cup plus 2 TBSP water, divided
- 1 cup granulated Swerve Sweetener
- 2 tsp lemon zest
- ¼ tsp salt
- 4 large egg yolks
- 1/3 cup lemon juice
- 3 TBSP butter
- ½ tsp xanthan gum
- 1 TBSP grassfed gelatin (can use 1 envelope Knox gelatin)

Crust

1. Preheat oven to 325°F.
2. Combine almond flour, coconut flour, arrowroot starch, sweetener, xanthan gum, and salt in the bowl of a food processor. Pulse to combine.
3. Sprinkle surface with butter pieces and pulse until mixture resembles coarse crumbs.
4. With processor running on low, add ice water, one tablespoon at a time until dough begins to clump together.

5. Place a large piece of parchment on work surface and dust liberally with additional almond flour. Turn out dough and pat into a circle. Sprinkle with more almond flour and cover with another large piece of parchment.

6. Roll out carefully into an 11-inch circle. Remove top layer of parchment. Place a 9-inch pie pan upside down on crust and then carefully flip both over so crust is lying in the pie pan. Remove parchment. (Alternatively, you can skip rolling out the pastry and simply press the crust into the bottom and up the sides of the pan.)

7. You may get some cracking and tears. Simply use small pieces of pastry from the overhang to patch them up. Crimp the edges of the crust and prick all over with a fork.

8. Bake crust 12 minutes, then remove and let cool.

Lemon Filling

1. In a medium saucepan over medium heat, combine 1 cup of the water, sweetener, lemon zest, and salt. Bring to just a boil, whisking frequently, until sweetener dissolves.

2. In a medium bowl, whisk egg yolks until smooth. Slowly add about ½ cup of the water to the egg yolks, whisking constantly. Then gradually whisk the egg yolks back into the pan and lower the heat to low. Cook for one minute more, stirring continuously.

3. Stir in lemon juice and butter and whisk until smooth. Sprinkle surface with xanthan gum and whisk vigorously to combine.

4. In a small bowl, stir together the remaining two tablespoons of water and the gelatin. Let sit two minutes until gelled, then stir into hot lemon mixture, whisking until well combined. Cover and set aside while making the meringue.

Meringue Topping

In a large bowl, beat egg whites with cream of tartar and salt until frothy. With beaters going, slowly add sweeteners and vanilla extract and continue to beat until stiff peaks form.

To Assemble

1. Preheat oven to 300°F.

2. Pour warm filling into crust. Dollop with meringue and spread right to the edges so that the meringue meets the crust. Swirl the top with the back of a spoon.

3. Bake 20 minutes or until meringue topping is golden and just barely firm to the touch. Remove and let pie cool 20 minutes, then refrigerate at least three hours to set.

Grasshopper Mousse Pie

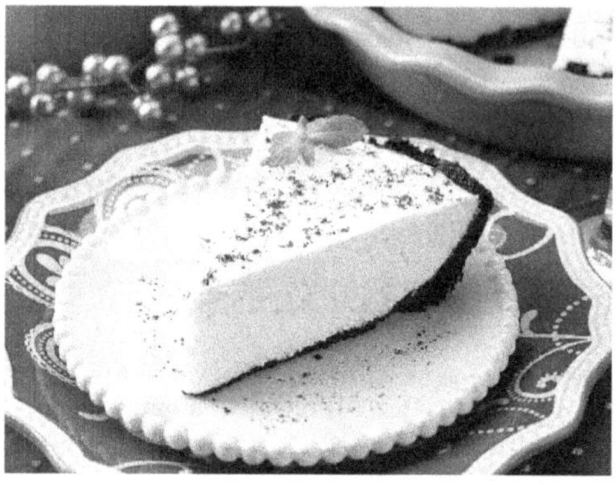

Calories: 261

Fat: 25 g

Carbohydrates: 5 g

Protein: 3 g

Prep Time: 20 minutes

Servings: 12

No-Bake Chocolate Pie Crust

- ¾ cup unsweetened shredded coconut
- ¼ cup unsweetened cocoa powder
- ½ cup sunflower seeds raw, unsalted
- 4 TBSP butter, softened
- ¼ tsp salt
- ¼ cup Swerve confectioners

Filling

- ½ cup water
- 1 tsp gelatin
- 5 oz avocado, mashed
- 8 oz cream cheese, softened
- 1 tsp peppermint extract
- 1 tsp peppermint liquid stevia
- Pinch of salt
- 1 cup heavy cream

Crust

1. Combine all ingredients into a food processor and blend just enough to combine. Don't over-blend or you will have the texture of peanut butter.
2. Taste crust to see if you need more salt or sweetness.
3. Using your fingers, spread and mold crust onto bottom and sides of pie plate. Set aside.

Filling

1. Pour the water into a small saucepan and sprinkle the gelatin on top.
2. Turn on low heat, stirring constantly until gelatin is dissolved. Let cool.
3. Place the avocado, cream cheese, peppermint extract, stevia, and salt into a stand mixer and blend on high until smooth.
4. Taste and adjust sweetness if needed.
5. Pour in heavy cream in another bowl and use an electric mixer to blend on high until soft peaks form. Fold into the cream cheese mixture.
6. Gradually pour in the cooled gelatin and stir until combined.
7. Pour filling into pie crust.
8. Refrigerate at least two hours, loosely covered or up to one day.
9. When ready to serve, add optional chocolate drizzle if desired.

Peanut Butter Molten Lava Cakes

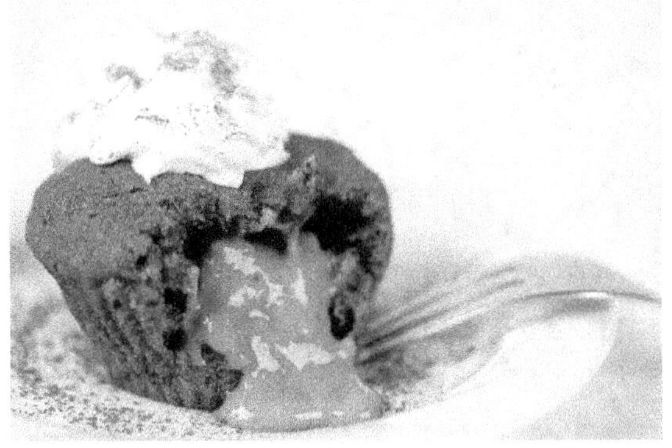

| Ingredients | Calories: 390
Fat: 35 g
Carbohydrates: 6 g
Protein: 10 g | Cook Time: 20 minutes
Servings: 4 |

- ¼ cup butter
- ¼ cup peanut butter
- 2 TBSP coconut oil
- 6 TBSP powdered Swerve Sweetener
- 2 large eggs
- 2 large egg yolks
- ½ tsp vanilla extract
- 6 TBSP almond flour
- Low-carb chocolate sauce

1. Preheat oven to 350°F and grease 4 small (about ½ cup capacity each) ramekins very well. I used both butter AND coconut oil spray.
2. In a medium-sized microwave safe bowl, combine butter, peanut butter, and coconut oil. Cook on high in 30-second increments until melted. Stir together until smooth.
3. Whisk in powdered sweetener until smooth. Whisk in eggs, egg yolks, and vanilla extract. Then whisk in almond flour until smooth.
4. Divide batter among prepared ramekins and bake 12 to 15 minutes, until sides are set but the center still jiggles a bit. Remove and let cool a few minutes.
5. Run a sharp knife around the inside of the ramekin to loosen the cakes. Cover each with an upside-down plate and flip over to turn the cake out onto the plate (you may need to give it one good shake, holding the plate and ramekin together tightly).
6. Drizzle with low-carb chocolate sauce and serve immediately.

Texas Sheet Cake

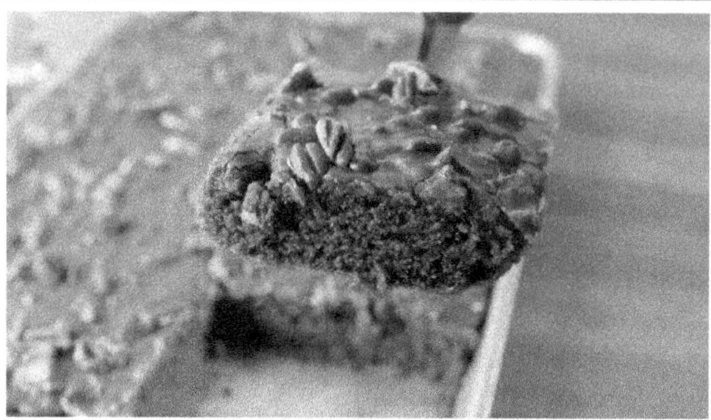

Calories: 230
Fat: 20 g
Carbohydrates: 6 g
Protein: 6 g

Cook Time:30 minutes
Servings:10

Cake

- 2 cups almond flour
- ¾ cup Swerve Sweetener
- 1/3 cup coconut flour
- 1/3 cup unflavoured whey protein powder
- 1 TBSP baking powder
- ½ tsp salt
- ½ cup butter
- ½ cup water
- ¼ cup cocoa powder
- 3 large eggs
- 1 tsp vanilla extract
- ¼ cup heavy cream
- ¼ cup water

Frosting

- ½ cup butter
- ¼ cup cocoa powder
- ¼ cup cream
- ¼ cup water
- 1 tsp vanilla extract
- 1 ½ cups powdered Swerve Sweetener
- ¼ tsp xanthan gum
- ¾ cup chopped pecans

Cake

1. Preheat oven to 325°F and grease a 10x15-inch rimmed sheet pan very well.
2. In a large bowl, whisk together the almond flour, sweetener, coconut flour, protein powder, baking powder, and salt. Break up any clumps with the back of a fork.
3. In a medium saucepan over medium heat, combine the butter, water, and cocoa powder, stirring until melted. Bring to a boil and then remove from heat. Add to the bowl.
4. Add eggs, vanilla extract, cream, and water, and stir until well combined. Spread in prepared baking pan.
5. Bake 15 to 20 minutes, until cake is set and a tester inserted in the center comes out clean. Drizzle with low-carb chocolate sauce and serve immediately.

Pecan Pie Cheesecake

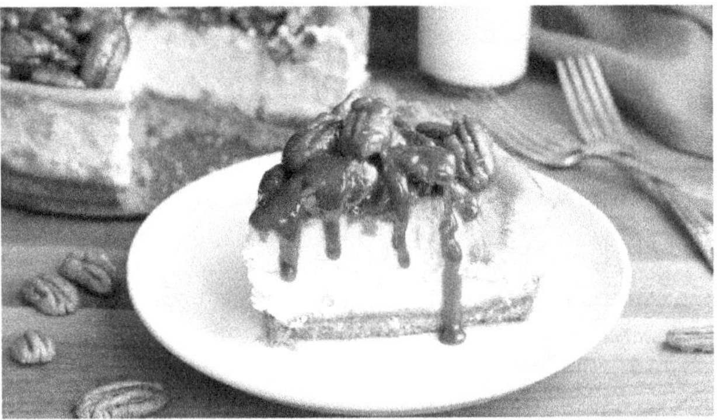

Ingredients

Calories: 340
Fat: 30 g
Carbohydrates: 5 g
Protein: 6 g

Cook Time:35 minutes
Servings: 10

Crust

- ¾ cup almond flour
- 2 TBSP powdered Swerve Sweetener
- Pinch of salt
- 2 TBSP melted butter

Pecan Pie Filling

- ¼ cup butter
- 1/3 cup powdered Swerve Sweetener
- 1 tsp Yacon syrup or molasses (optional, for color and flavor
- 1 tsp caramel extract or vanilla extract
- 2 TBSP heavy whipping cream
- 1 large egg
- ¼ tsp salt
- ½ cup chopped pecans

Cheesecake Filling

- 12 oz cream cheese, softened
- 5 TBSP powdered Swerve Sweetener
- 1 large egg
- ¼ cup heavy whipping cream
- ½ tsp vanilla extract

Topping

- 2 TBSP butter
- 2 ½ TBSP powdered Swerve Sweetener
- ½ tsp Yacon syrup or molasses
- ½ tsp caramel extract or vanilla extract
- 1 TBSP heavy whipping cream
- Whole toasted pecans for garnish

Crust

1. In a medium bowl, whisk together the almond flour, sweetener, and salt. Stir in the melted butter until the mixture begins to clump together.
2. Press into the bottom and partway up the sides of a 7-inch springform pan. Place in the freezer while making the pecan pie filling.

Pecan Pie Filling

1. In a small saucepan over low heat, melt the butter. Add the sweetener and Yacon syrup and whisk until combined, then stir in the extract and heavy whipping cream.

2. Add the egg and continue to cook over low heat until the mixture thickens (this should only take a minute or so). Immediately remove from heat and stir in the pecans and salt.

3. Spread mixture over the bottom of the crust.

Cheesecake Filling

1. Beat the cream cheese until smooth, then beat in the sweetener. Beat in the egg, whipping cream, and vanilla extract.

2. Pour this mixture over the pecan pie filling and spread to the edges.

To Bake

1. Wrap the bottom of the springform pan tightly in a large piece of foil. Place a piece of paper towel over the top of the springform pan (not touching the cheesecake) and then wrap foil around the top as well. Your whole pan should be mostly covered in foil to keep out excess moisture.

2. Place the rack that came with your Instant Pot or pressure cooker into the bottom. Pour a cup of water into the bottom.

3. Carefully lower the wrapped cheesecake pan onto the rack (there are ways to do this with a sling made out of tin foil but I didn't bother with that).

4. Close the lid and set the Instant Pot to manual mode for 30 minutes on high. Once the cooking time is complete, let the pressure to release naturally (do not vent it).

5. Lift out the cheesecake and let it cool to room temperature, and then refrigerate for three or four hours, or even overnight.

Topping

1. In a small saucepan over low heat, melt the butter. Add the sweetener and Yacon syrup and whisk until combined, then stir in the extract and heavy whipping cream.

2. Drizzle over the chilled cheesecake and garnish with toasted pecans.

Chocolate Walnut Torte

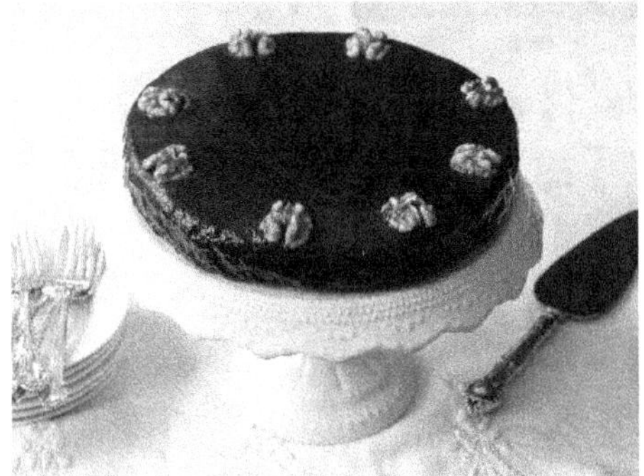

Calories: 343

Fat: 31 g

Carbohydrates: 9 g

Protein: 9 g

Cook Time: 30 minutes

Servings: 1

Torte

- 1 ½ cup walnuts
- ¾ cup Swerve Sweetener
- ¼ cup cocoa powder
- 1 tsp espresso powder (optional, enhances chocolate flavor)
- ½ tsp baking powder
- ¼ tsp salt
- ½ cup butter
- 4 oz unsweetened chocolate
- 5 large eggs
- ½ tsp vanilla extract
  ½ cup almond milk

Glaze

- ½ cup whipping cream
- 2 ½ oz sugar-free dark chocolate chopped
- 1/3 cup walnut pieces

Torte

1. Preheat oven to 325°F and grease a 9-inch round baking pan. Line the bottom with parchment paper and grease the paper.
2. In a food processor, process walnuts until finely ground. Add sweetener, cocoa powder, espresso powder, baking powder, and salt, and pulse a few times to combine.
3. In a large saucepan set over low heat, melt butter and chocolate together until smooth. Remove from heat and whisk in eggs and vanilla extract. Add almond milk and whisk until mixture smooths out. Stir in walnut mixture until well combined.
4. Spread batter in prepared baking pan and bake about 30 minutes, until edges are set but center still looks slightly wet. Let cool 15 minutes in pan, then invert onto a wire rack to cool completely. Remove parchment paper.

Glaze

1. In a small saucepan over medium heat, bring cream to just a simmer. Remove from heat and add chopped chocolate. Let sit to melt five minutes, then whisk until smooth.
2. Cool another ten minutes, then pour the glaze over the cake, smoothing the sides. Sprinkle top with walnut pieces and chill until chocolate is firm, about 30 minutes.

Classic New York Keto Cheesecake

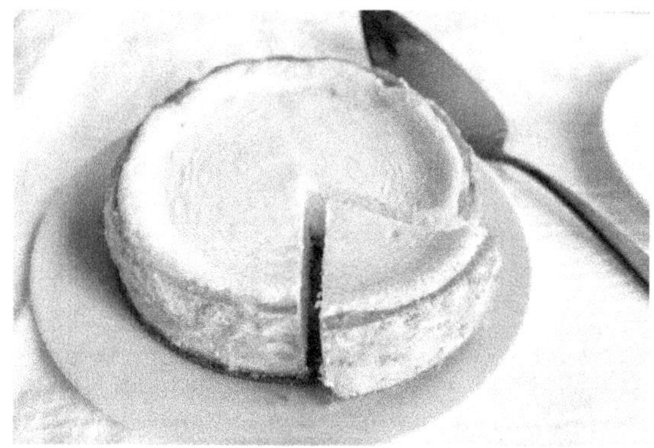

Ingredients	Calories: 284	Cook Time: 1 hour 30 minutes
	Fat: 24 g	
	Carbohydrates: 3 g	Servings: 12
	Protein: 5 g	

- 24 oz cream cheese, softened
- 5 TBSP unsalted butter, softened
- 1 cup powdered Swerve Sweetener
- 3 large eggs, room temperature
- ¾ cup sour cream, room temperature
- 2 tsp grated lemon zest
- 1 ½ tsp vanilla extract

1. Preheat the oven to 300°F and generously grease a 9-inch springform pan. Cut a circle of parchment to fit the bottom of the pan and grease the paper. Wrap two pieces of aluminum foil around the outside of the pan to cover the bottom and most of the way up the sides.

2. In a large bowl, beat the cream cheese and butter until smooth, then beat in the sweetener until well combined. Add the eggs, one at a time, beating after each addition. Clean the beaters and scrape down the sides of the bowl as needed.

3. Add the sour cream, lemon zest, and vanilla extract and beat until the batter is smooth and well combined. Pour into the prepared springform pan and smooth the top.

4. Set the pan inside a roasting pan large enough to prevent the sides from touching. Place the roasting pan in the oven and carefully pour boiling water into the roasting pan until it reaches halfway up the sides of the springform pan.

5. Bake 70 to 90 minutes, until the cheesecake is mostly set but still jiggles just a little in the center when shaken. Remove the roasting pan from the one, then carefully remove the springform pan from the water bath. Let cool to room temperature.

6. Run a sharp knife around the edges of the cake to loosen, then release the sides of the pan. Refrigerate for at least four hours before serving.

Bread

If you're on a ketogenic diet, you don't have to give up your addiction to freshly baked bread. Here you will find recipes that will help you enjoy bread while maintaining your keto lifestyle.

Storage of bread. When the baked bread has cooled, wrap the loaf in plastic wrap or a freezer bag and place it in the refrigerator or freezer. Baked bread can be stored in the freezer for up to six months. To defrost the bread, remove it from the freezer, partially unfold the loaf, and leave to stand at room temperature. If you want to drop the bread warm after refrigeration or freezing, wrap the bread in aluminum foil and bake in an oven preheated to 300°F for 10–15 minutes.

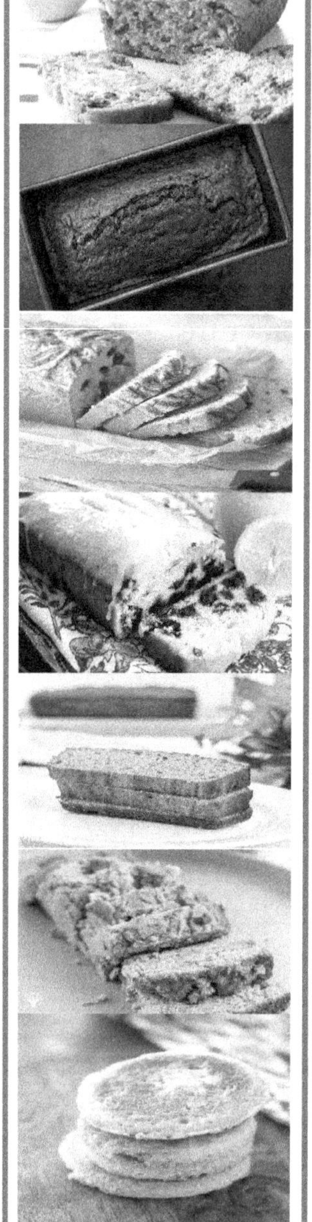

Cranberry Bread

Chocolate Zucchini Bread

Cinnamon Almond Flour Bread

Blueberry English Muffin Bread

Pumpkin Bread

Zucchini Bread with Walnuts

90-Second Microwavable Keto Bread

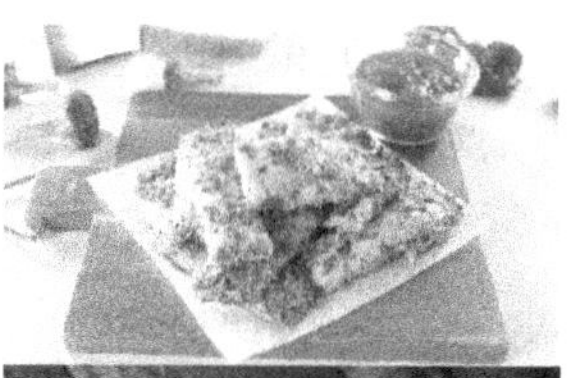

Broccoli Cheesy Bread

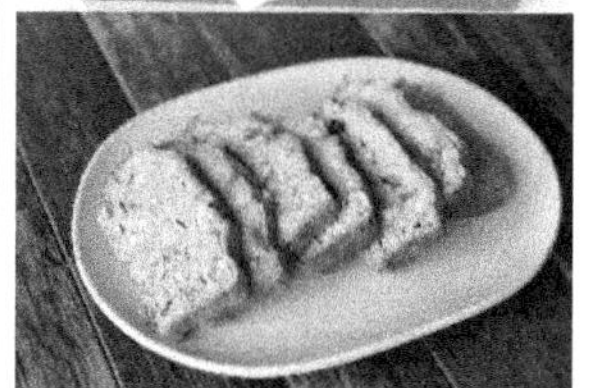

Sundried Tomato Low Carb Bread

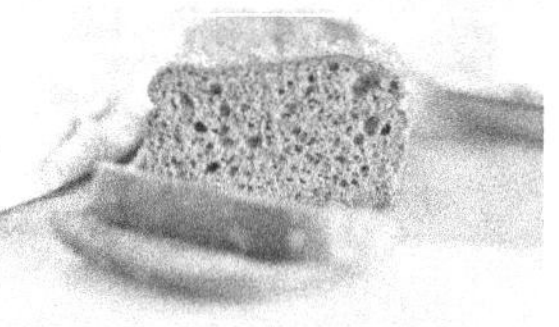

Keto Bread

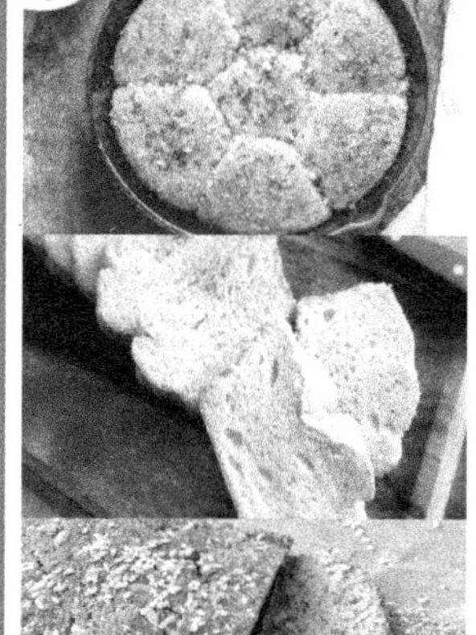

Garlic Butter Keto Bread

Collagen Keto Bread

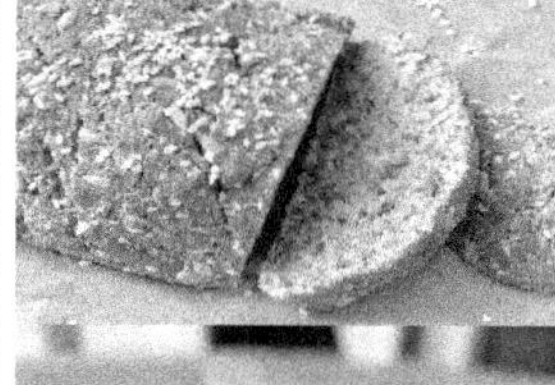

Keto Bread without Eggs

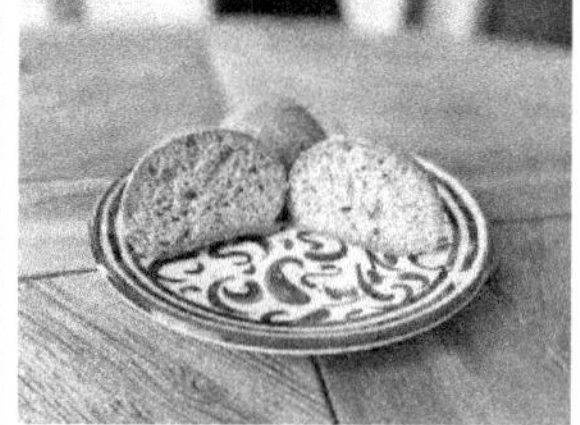

5-Minute Gluten-Free Keto Bread Rolls

Cranberry Bread

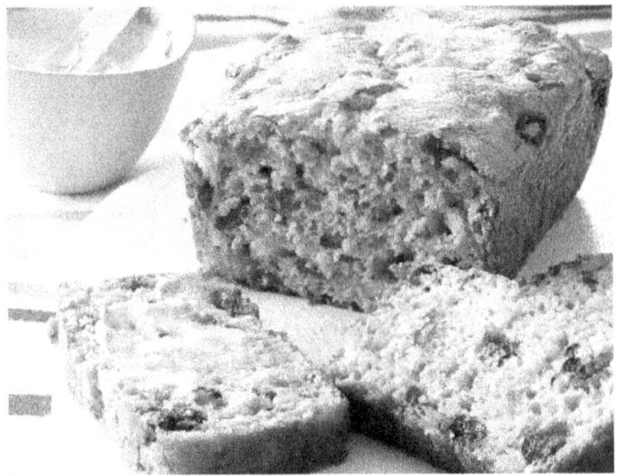

	Calories: 180	Cook Time: 1 hour 15
Ingredients	Fat: 15 g	minutes
	Carbohydrates: 7 g	Servings: 12
	Protein: 7 g	

- 2 cups almond flour
- ½ cup powdered erythritol or Swerve, (see Note)
- ½ tsp Steviva stevia powder (see Note)
- 1 ½ tsp baking powder
- ½ tsp baking soda
- 1 tsp salt
- 4 TBSP unsalted butter, melted (or coconut oil)
- 1 tsp blackstrap molasses (optional [for brown sugar flavor])
- 4 large eggs at room temperature
- ½ cup coconut milk
- 1 bag cranberries, 12 oz

1. Preheat oven to 350°F; grease a 9-by-5-inch loaf pan and set aside.
2. In a large bowl, whisk together flour, erythritol, stevia, baking powder, baking soda, and salt; set aside.
3. In a medium bowl, combine butter, molasses, eggs, and coconut milk.
4. Mix dry mixture into wet mixture until well combined.
5. Fold in cranberries. Pour batter into prepared pan.
6. Bake until a toothpick inserted in the center of the loaf comes clean, about 1 hour and 15 minutes.
7. Transfer pan to a wire rack; let bread cool 15 minutes before removing from pan.

Chocolate Zucchini Bread

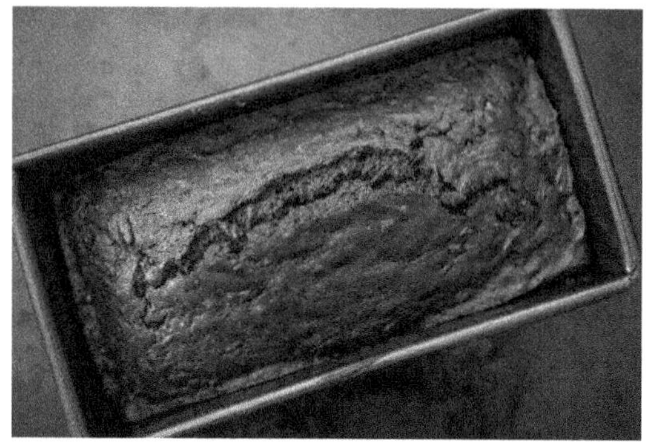

Calories: 185
Fat: 17 g
Carbohydrates: 6 g
Protein: 5

Cook Time: 50 minutes
Servings: 12

Dry Ingredients
- 1 ½ cup almond flour (170 g)
- ¼ cup unsweetened cocoa powder (25 g)
- 1 ½ tsp baking soda
- 2 tsp ground cinnamon
- ¼ tsp sea salt
- ½ cup sugar-free crystal sweetener (Monk fruit or erythritol) (100 g) or coconut sugar if refined sugar-free

Wet Ingredients
- 1 cup zucchini, finely grated measure packed, discard juice/liquid if there is some (about 2 small zucchini)
- 1 large egg
- ¼ cup + 2 TBSP canned coconut cream (100 ml)
- ¼ cup extra virgin coconut oil, melted (60ml)
- 1 tsp vanilla extract
- 1 tsp apple cider vinegar

Filling (optional)
- ½ cup sugar-free chocolate chips
- ½ cup chopped walnuts (or nuts you like)

1. Preheat oven to 180°C (375°F). Line a baking loaf pan (9 inches x 5 inches) with parchment paper. Set aside.
2. Remove both extremities of the zucchinis, keep skin on.
3. Finely grate the zucchini using a vegetable grater. Measure the amount needed in a measurement cup. Make sure you press/pack them firmly for a precise measure and to squeeze out any liquid from the grated zucchini, I usually don't have any! If you do, discard the liquid or keep for another recipe.
4. In a large mixing bowl, stir all the dry ingredients together: almond flour, unsweetened cocoa powder, sugar-free crystal sweetener, cinnamon, sea salt, and baking soda. Set aside.
5. Add all the wet ingredients into the dry ingredients: grated zucchini, coconut oil, coconut cream, vanilla, egg, apple cider vinegar.
6. Stir to combine all the ingredients together.
7. Stir in the chopped nuts and sugar-free chocolate chips.
8. Transfer the chocolate bread batter into the prepared loaf pan.
9. Bake 50–55 minutes—you may want to cover the bread loaf with a piece of foil after 40 minutes to avoid the top to darken too much, up to you.
10. The bread will stay slightly moist in the middle and firm up after fully cooled down.
11. Transfer pan to a wire rack; let bread cool 15 minutes before removing from pan.

Cinnamon Almond Flour Bread

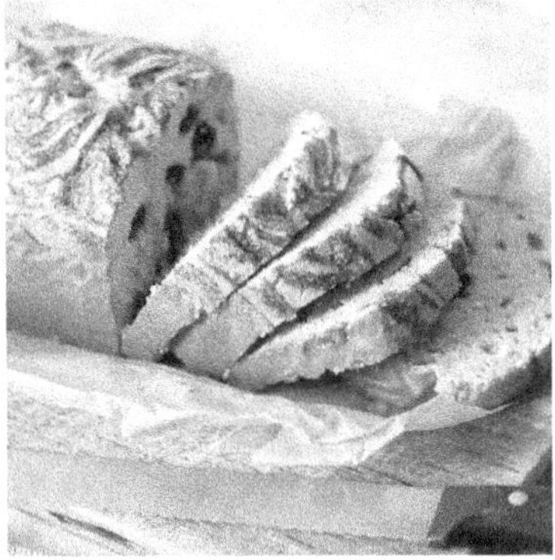

Calories: 221	Cook Time: 30 minutes
Fat: 15 g	
Carbohydrates: 10 g	Servings: 8
Protein: 9 g	

Ingredients

- 2 cups fine blanched almond flour (I use Bob's Red Mill)
- 2 TBSP coconut flour
- ½ tsp sea salt
- 1 tsp baking soda
- ¼ cup flaxseed meal or chia meal (ground chia or flaxseed, see notes for how to make your own)
- 5 eggs and 1 egg white whisked together
- 1.5 tsp apple cider vinegar or lemon juice
- 2 TBSP maple syrup or honey
- 2–3 TBSP of clarified butter (melted) or coconut oil (divided). Vegan butter also works.
- 1 TBSP cinnamon, plus extra for topping
- Optional: Chia seeds to sprinkle on top before baking

1. Preheat oven to 350°F. Line an 8×4-inch bread pan with parchment paper at the bottom and grease the sides.
2. In a large bowl, mix together your almond flour, coconut flour, salt, baking soda, flaxseed meal or chia meal, and ½ tablespoon of cinnamon.
3. In another small bowl, whisk together your eggs and egg white. Then add in your maple syrup (or honey), apple cider vinegar, and melted butter (1.5 to 2 tablespoons).
4. Mix wet ingredients into dry. Be sure to remove any clumps that might have occurred from the almond flour or coconut flour.
5. Pour batter into a your greased loaf pan.
6. Bake at 350°F for 30–35 minutes, until a toothpick inserted into center of loaf comes out clean. Mine came to around 35 minutes, but I am at altitude.
7. Remove from the oven.
8. Next, whisk together the other 1 to 2 tablespoons of melted butter (or oil) and mix it with ½ tablespoon of cinnamon. Brush this on top of your cinnamon almond flour bread.
9. Cool and serve, or store for later.
10. Transfer pan to a wire rack; let bread cool 15 minutes before removing from pan.

Blueberry English Muffin Bread

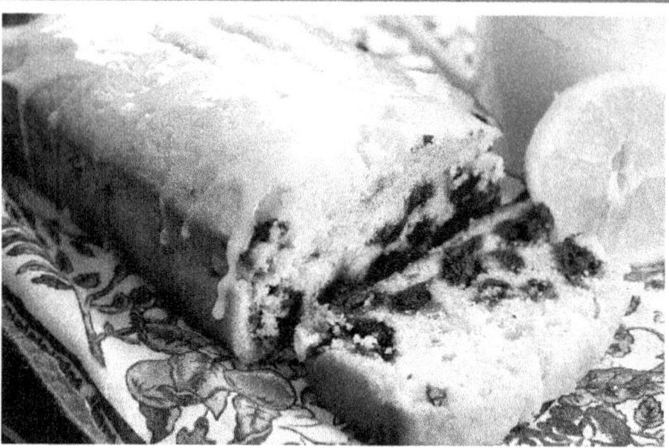

Calories: 156

Fat: 13 g

Carbohydrates: 4 g

Protein: 5 g

Cook Time: 45 minutes

Servings: 12

- ½ cup almond butter, cashew, or peanut butter
- ¼ cup butter ghee or coconut oil
- ½ cup almond flour
  ½ tsp salt
- 5 eggs and 1 egg white whisked together
- 2 tsp baking powder
- ½ cup almond milk, unsweetened
- 5 eggs, beaten
- ½ cup blueberries

1. Preheat oven to 350°F.
2. In a microwavable bowl melt nut butter and butter together for 30 seconds; stir until combined well.
3. In a large bowl, whisk almond flour, salt, and baking powder together. Pour the nut butter mixture into the large bowl and stir to combine.
4. Whisk the almond milk and eggs together then pour into the bowl and stir well.
5. Drop in fresh blueberries or break apart frozen blueberries and gently stir into the batter.
6. Line a loaf pan with parchment paper and lightly grease the parchment paper as well.
7. Pour the batter into the loaf pan and bake 45 minutes or until a toothpick in center comes out clean.
8. Cool for about 30 minutes then remove from pan.
9. Slice and toast each slice before serving ½ cup chopped walnuts (or nuts you like)

Pumpkin Bread

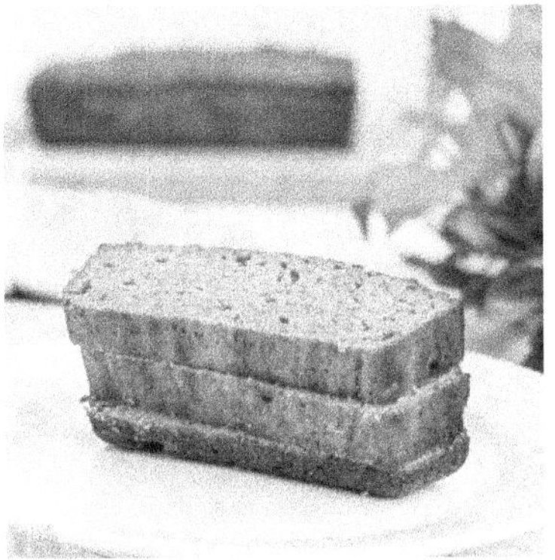

Calories: 165	Cook Time: 45 minutes
Fat: 14 g	
Carbohydrates: 6 g	Servings: 10
Protein: 5 g	

- ½ cup butter, softened
- 2/3 cup erythritol sweetener, like Swerve
- 4 eggs, large
- ¾ cup pumpkin puree, canned
- 1 tsp vanilla extract
- 1 ½ cup almond flour
- ½ cup coconut flour
- 4 tsp baking powder
- 1 tsp cinnamon
- ½ tsp nutmeg
- ¼ tsp ginger
- 1/8 tsp cloves
- ½ tsp salt

1. Preheat the oven to 350°F. Grease a 9"x5" loaf pan, and line with parchment paper.
2. In a large mixing bowl, cream the butter and sweetener together until light and fluffy.
3. Add the eggs, one at a time, and mix well to combine.
4. Add the pumpkin puree and vanilla, and mix well to combine.
5. In a separate bowl, stir together the almond flour, coconut flour, baking powder, cinnamon, nutmeg, ginger, cloves, and salt. Break up any lumps of almond flour or coconut flour.
6. Add the dry ingredients to the wet ingredients, and stir to combine. (Optionally, add up to ½ cup of mix-ins, like chopped nuts or chocolate chips.)
7. Pour the batter into the prepared loaf pan. Bake for 45–55 minutes, or until a toothpick inserted into the center of the loaf comes out clean.
8. If the bread is browning too quickly, you can cover the pan with a piece of aluminum foil.

Zucchini Bread with Walnuts

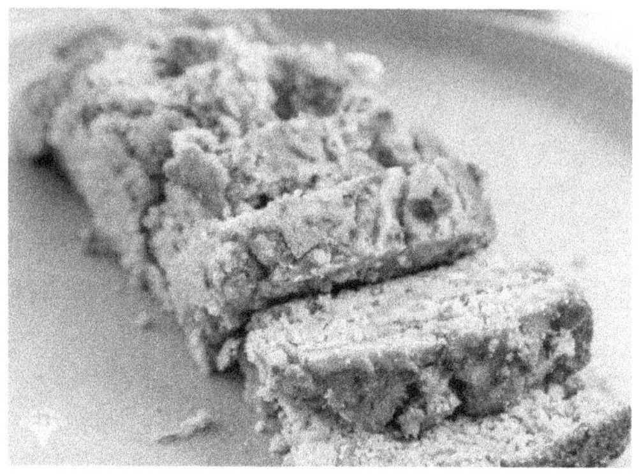

Calories: 200
Fat: 18 g
Carbohydrates: 3 g
Protein: 5 g

Cook Time: 60 minutes
Servings: 10

- 3 large eggs
- ½ cup olive oil
- 1 tsp vanilla extract
- 2 ½ cups almond flour
- 1 ½ cups erythritol
- ½ tsp salt
- 1 ½ tsp baking powder
- ½ tsp nutmeg
- 1 tsp ground cinnamon
- ¼ tsp ground ginger
- 1 cup grated zucchini
- ½ cup chopped walnuts

1. Preheat oven to 350°F. Whisk together the eggs, oil, and vanilla extract. Set to the side.
2. In another bowl, mix together the almond flour, erythritol, salt, baking powder, nutmeg, cinnamon, and ginger. Set to the side.
3. Using a cheesecloth or paper towel, take the zucchini and squeeze out the excess water.
4. Then, whisk the zucchini into the bowl with the eggs.
5. Slowly add the dry ingredients into the egg mixture using a hand mixer until fully blended.
6. Lightly spray a 9x5 loaf pan, and spoon in the zucchini bread mixture.
7. Then, spoon in the chopped walnuts on top of the zucchini bread. Press walnuts into the batter using a spatula.
8. Bake for 60–70 minutes at 350°F or until the walnuts on top look browned.

90-Second Microwavable Keto Bread

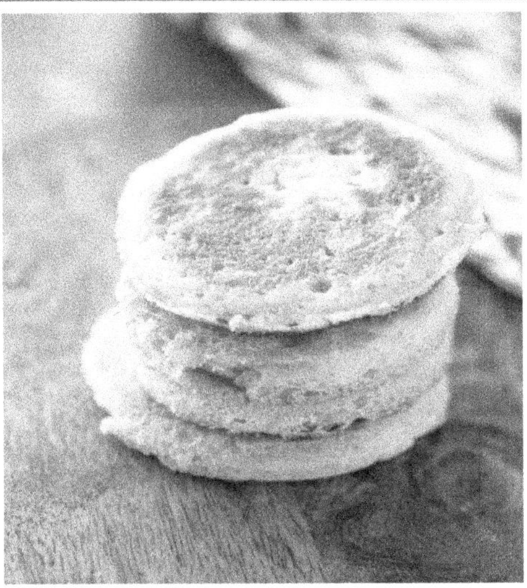

Calories: 170
Fat: 15 g
Carbohydrates: 3 g
Protein: 5 g

Cook Time: 15 minutes
Servings: 2

- 3 tablespoons almond flour or 1 tablespoon coconut flour
- 1 tablespoon butter or oil
- 1 medium/large egg
- ½ teaspoon double-acting baking powder

1. Melt butter in a microwave-safe bowl or ramekin. Add the almond flour, egg, and baking powder to the butter. Beat with a fork until completely mix.

2. Microwave for about 90 seconds, until firm. Run a knife along the edge and flip over a plate to release. Slice in half, then toast in the toaster or a skillet.

3. To Bake: Preheat oven to 375°F. Bake in a ramekin for 10–12 minutes or until cooked through.

Broccoli Cheesy Bread

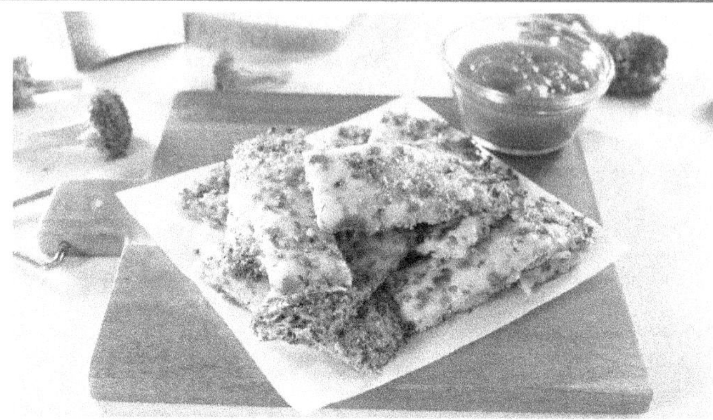

Calories: 258
Fat: 17 g
Carbohydrates: 4 g
Protein: 17 g

Cook Time: 25 minutes
Servings: 4

- 3 cups broccoli
- 1 large egg
- ¼ cup Parmesan cheese freshly grated
- 1 ½ cup cheddar cheese shredded
- 2 tsp almond flour
- ½ tsp garlic powder
- salt
- black pepper

1. Wash and dry your fresh broccoli bunch. Discard all of the leaves before chopping into chunks. Make sure to chop enough chunks for 3 cups.
2. Transfer the chopped broccoli pieces into a food processor. Continue pulsing until you get rice-size bits.
3. Set the microwave to "cooking." Leave the broccoli rice in the microwave for a minute and a half.
4. Crack the egg in a bowl. Add the garlic, cheddar cheese, and almond flour together with the riced broccoli. Beat with a spoon until combined. Season with a dash of pepper and salt.
5. Pat the mixture into a baking tray covered with waxed paper. Cover all sides of the tray evenly.
6. Sprinkle a generous amount of Parmesan cheese on top. Put in the oven for 10 minutes. The oven should be set at 300°F.
7. Take the tray out of the oven. Top with half a cup of cheddar cheese. Rebake for five more minutes to melt the cheese.
8. Once ready, remove from the heat. Allow cooling for around five minutes then remove the paper.
9. Cut into rectangular shapes and enjoy!

Sundried Tomato Low-Carb Bread

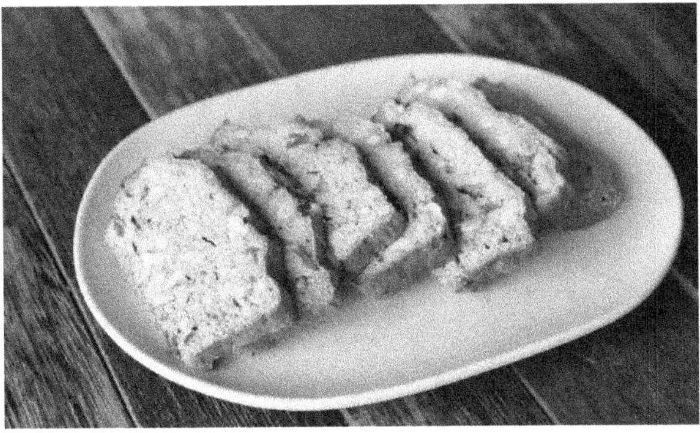

Calories: 200
Fat: 12 g
Carbohydrates: 4 g
Protein: 12 g

Cook Time: 50 minutes
Servings: 6

- 8 eggs
- 10 sundried tomatoes chopped
- ½ cup butter, melted
- ½ cup pine nuts
- ½ cup sesame seeds
- ¼ cup coconut flour
- ¼ cup chia seeds
- ¼ cup fresh basil chopped (optional)
- 1 TBSP onion flakes
- salt and pepper

1. Preheat oven to 180°C (350°F) and line a 20 x 10cm (8 x 4-inch) loaf tin with baking paper.
2. In a food processor, mix the eggs and butter on high speed until smooth (about two minutes).
3. Add the sesame seeds, coconut flour, chia seeds, basil, onion flakes, salt, and pepper. Whiz again on medium speed until combined.
4. Transfer the mixture into a bowl, add the pine nuts and sundried tomatoes and mix well.
5. Spoon the mixture into the prepared loaf tin and place it in the oven for 40 minutes or until golden-brown on top.
6. Allow to cool before slicing.

Keto Bread

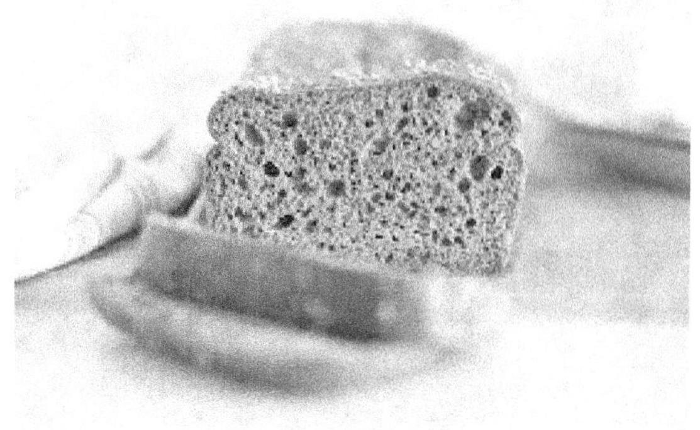

Calories: 200
Fat: 18 g
Carbohydrates:22g
Protein: 12 g

Cook Time:60
minutes
Servings: 6

- 1 ¼ cups (5oz/143g) almond flour
- 5 tablespoons (1 1/2oz/44g) psyllium husk powder
- 2 teaspoons baking powder
- 1 teaspoon salt
- 2 teaspoons apple cider vinegar
- 1 cup (8floz/225ml) boiling water
- 3 egg whites

1. Preheat your oven to 350°F (180°C), then butter and line a 9x5-inch loaf tin with parchment paper. Set aside.
2. In a large bowl, combine the almond flour, psyllium husk*, baking powder, and salt.
3. Add the egg whites and apple cider vinegar to the dry ingredients with an electric mixer on medium speed until a paste-like dough is formed.
4. While mixing on low speed, stream in the boiling water. Turn the speed up to high and mix for about 30 seconds, or until the dough forms an elastic Play-Doh-like mixture. Be careful not to over-mix!
5. Transfer the dough to the prepared baking tin and smooth the top. Lastly, sprinkle over the sesame seeds.
6. Bake the bread for 55–65 minutes or until the top has risen and puffed up like a traditional sandwich loaf.
7. Remove the bread from the oven and allow to cool slightly before transferring to a cooling rack. (Note: this bread has a tendency to fall or deflate a little once out of the oven. Please see my update above the recipe.)
8. Once cooled, slice and enjoy! Store the bread covered at room temperature for two days. After two days, I suggest storing it in the fridge for no longer than another two days.

Garlic Butter Keto Bread

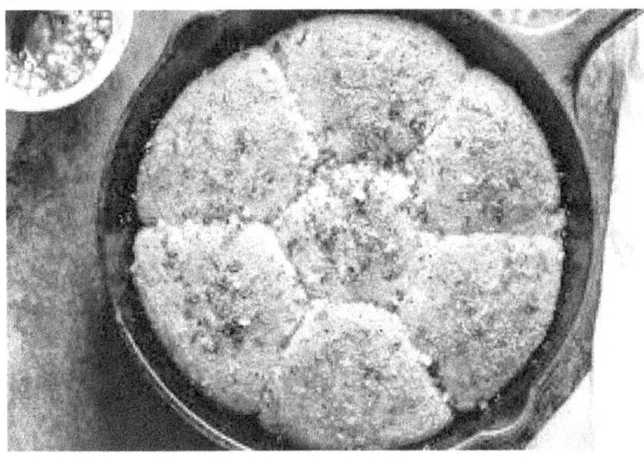

Calories: 258
Fat: 17 g
Carbohydrates: 4 g
Protein: 17 g

Cook Time:25 minutes
Servings: 4

Ingredients

Bread

- 2 ½ cups mozzarella, shredded
- 2 oz cream cheese
- 3 eggs
- 1 ½ cups almond flour (super-fine)
- 1 teaspoon baking powder
- 1/3 cup cooked bacon bits
- ½ cup grated Parmesan
- 1 teaspoon Italian seasoning
- 2 tsp almond flour
- ½ tsp garlic powder
- salt
- black pepper

The garlic butter sauce

- ¼ cup browned butter
- 4 garlic cloves, finely minced
- ½ cup fresh parsley, chopped

1. To make this garlic butter keto bread recipe – Grease a medium cast-iron skillet with oil, butter, or cooking spray and set aside. In a shallow plate, combine parmesan and Italian seasoning.
2. Melt mozzarella and cream cheese in a large bowl for one minute in the microwave. Mix well with a spatula until smooth.
3. Combine the melted cheese, eggs, baking powder, almond flour, and bacon. Mix until smooth.
4. Using a large cookie scoop, scoop dough and bread roll into the parmesan and Italian seasoning mix. Place each bread roll into the prepared cast-iron skillet. Sprinkle bread roll with more parmesan cheese. Place skillet in the refrigerator for 10 minutes. In the meantime, preheat your oven to 400°F (200°C).
5. Remove the cast-iron skillet from the refrigerator. Bake the garlic butter bread for 20 to 25 minutes, until golden-brown.
6. Brush the baked garlic butter keto bread generously with the garlic butter sauce and serve. Enjoy!

Collagen Keto Bread

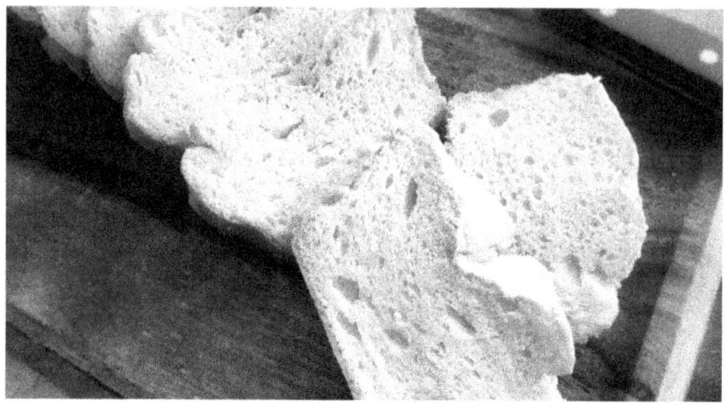

Calories: 225
Fat: 25 g
Carbohydrates: 4 g
Protein: 17 g

Cook Time: 30 minutes
Servings: 10

- ½ cup Perfect Keto Collagen (about 50g)
- 5 egg whites and yolks separated
- 6 TBSP coconut flour
- 3 TBSP coconut milk full-fat
- 1 tsp xanthan gum
- 2 tsp almond flour
- 1 tsp baking powder, keto-friendly
- 1 pinch sea salt
- 1 TBSP coconut oil melted (+ more for greasing)

1. Preheat the oven to 325°F.
2. In a bowl, combine all the dry ingredients.
3. In a small bowl, whisk together coconut milk, egg yolks, and melted coconut oil.
4. In another bowl, whip egg whites until peaks form.
5. Fold both dry and wet ingredients in the whipped egg whites bowl and mix until incorporated.
6. Brush your loaf dish (9x5x3-inch size) with coconut oil.
7. Pour the batter into a loaf dish and bake for 40 minutes.
8. Let cool completely and slice.
9. Remove the cast-iron skillet from the refrigerator. Bake the garlic butter bread for 20 to 25 minutes, until golden-brown.
10. Brush the baked garlic butter keto bread generously with the garlic butter sauce and serve. Enjoy!

Keto Bread without Eggs

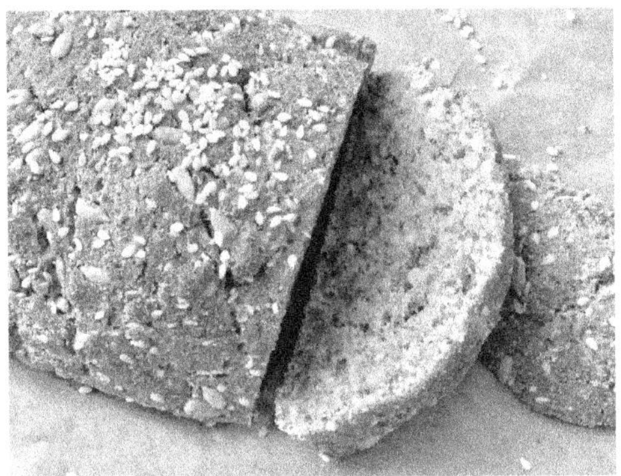

Calories: 225
Fat: 30 g
Carbohydrates: 80 g
Protein:17g

Cook Time:70 minutes
Servings: 14

DRY INGREDIENTS

- 2 ½ cup almond flour, not almond meal!
- ½ cup coconut flour
- 1/3 cup flaxseed meal
- 1/3 cup + 2 TBSP whole psyllium husk
- 1 TBSP baking powder
- ½ tablespoon salt

LIQUID INGREDIENTS

- 2 tablespoons extra virgin olive oil
- 1 teaspoon apple cider vinegar
- 2 cups lukewarm water - think bath temperature, 40°C/100°F

1. Preheat oven to 200°C (400°F). Line a 9 x 5-inch loaf pan with a piece of parchment paper. Slightly oil the paper to make sure the bread doesn't stick to the pan. Set aside.
2. In a large mixing bowl, add all the dry ingredients, whisk to combine.
3. Add the liquid ingredients; order doesn't matter. Combine with a spatula or spoon, then use your hand to knead the dough for about one or two minutes The batter is very moist at first, getting dryer as you go. After two minutes, it should come together easily to form a dough. If not too sticky, add more husk, ½ teaspoon at a time, knead for 30 seconds and see how it goes. The dough will always be a bit moist, but it shouldn't stick to your hands at all. If so, the bread will be too moist when baked.
4. Set aside 10 minutes to let the fiber fully absorb the liquid.
5. Shape the dough as you want your bread to look like when baked. I mean, you want a lovely round bun on top of your loaf. So shape a cylinder of dough that matches the length of the pan, but DO NOT press or flatten the top of your loaf, or you will end up with a more dense/tight crumb. Keep the top round shape; it's what will create a bread loaf that is soft and light with holes in the crumb.

6. Slightly rub your hand with water and massage the bread's surface to remove any holes and create a smooth surface.

7. Bake for 50–55 minutes in the center of the oven; fan-bake mode is the best.

8. After 50 minutes, prick the center of the loaf with a skewer to test. If it comes out clean, it is cooked. If not, it means the bread is still wet inside, cover the loaf pan with a piece of foil, reduce heat to 180°C (375°F), and keep baking for 20–30 minutes until cooked in the middle.

9. Lift the bread out of the pan using the parchment paper.

10. Fully cool down on a rack before slicing—at least three hours for best results.

11. Slice into 16 slices. Store in the fridge for up to five days or freeze up to three months in airtight containers.

5-Minute Gluten-Free Keto Bread Rolls

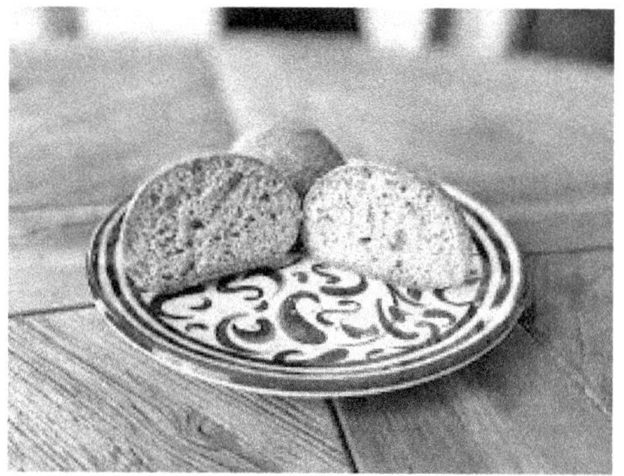

Ingredients	Calories: 642	Cook Time: 65
	Fat: 48 g	minutes
	Carbohydrates: 42 g	Servings: 6
	Protein: 30 g	

- ¾ cup almond flour* organic
- 2 ¾ TBSP psyllium husk* organic
- 2 tsp baking powder*
- 1 tsp salt* real salt
- 1 cup water boiling

- 3 egg whites* pastured
- 1 TBSP chia seeds* substitute with sesame seeds
- 1 splash apple cider vinegar* optional

1. Prepare a baking sheet and line with a silicone baking mat or parchment paper.
2. Preheat oven to 350°F
3. Fill a bowl with warm water.
4. Preheat oven to 350°F (180°C),
5. Add the dry ingredients (almond flour, psyllium husk, baking powder, and salt) into a bowl and mix by hand.

6.	Add the boiling water, egg whites, and an optional splash of apple cider vinegar.
7.	Mix by hand using a spatula.
8.	Moisten your hands, form six rolls, and place them on the baking sheet.
9.	Sprinkle the bread rolls with chia or sesame seeds.
10.	Place the baking sheet in the oven for 50–60 minutes.
11.	To check if they're done, carefully tap on one of the rolls to see if they sound hollow. If they do sound hollow, you can take them out and let them cool down.

Keto Chaffle

Keto waffles are a salvation for everyone who follows the keto diet. This is a great alternative to bread. Or a sweet treat. Keto waffles are very simple and versatile, and you only need a few common ingredients to make them.

Storage. Cooked waffles can be stored for up to three days at room temperature or for a week in the refrigerator. If you wrap them with aluminum foil, they will keep fresh. You can freeze keto waffles for up to three months and let them defrost at room temperature.

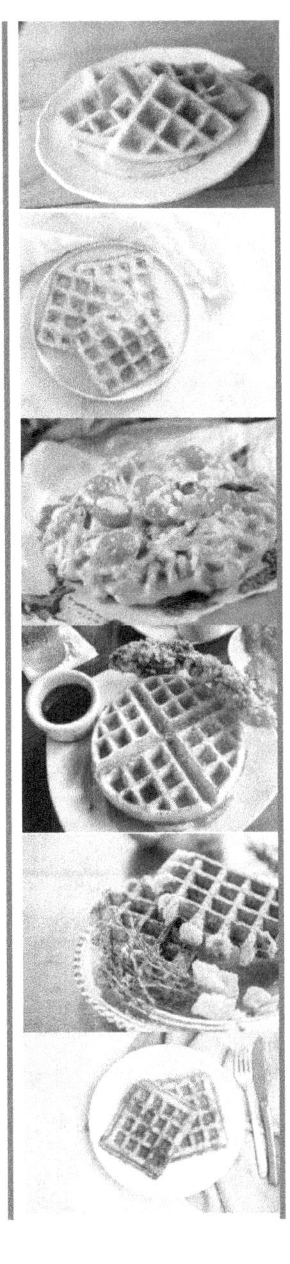

Cauliflower Chaffle

Parmesan and Garlic Chaffles

Pizza Chaffle

Buffalo Chicken Chaffle

Cheddar Chaffles

Egg and Mozzarella Chaffle

Jalapeno and Cheddar Chaffle

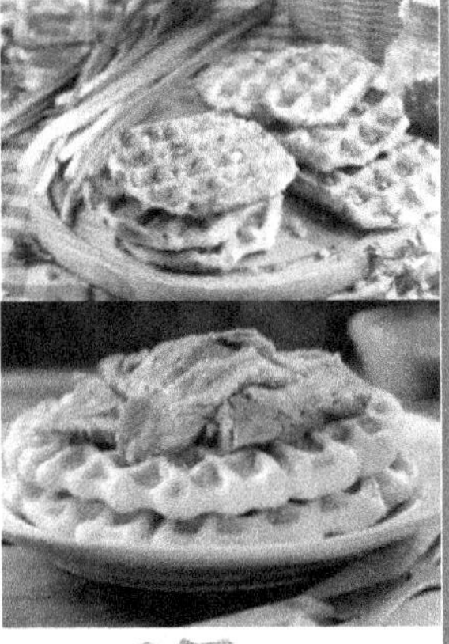

Beef and Onion Bun Chaffle

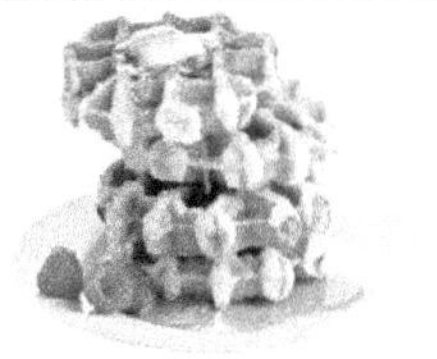

Belgian Chaffles

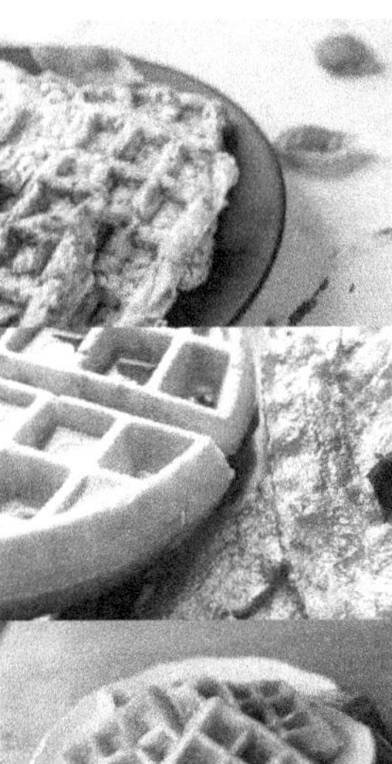

Broccoli and Cheese Chaffle

Bacon Chaffles

Cannabis Chaffles

Cauliflower Chaffle

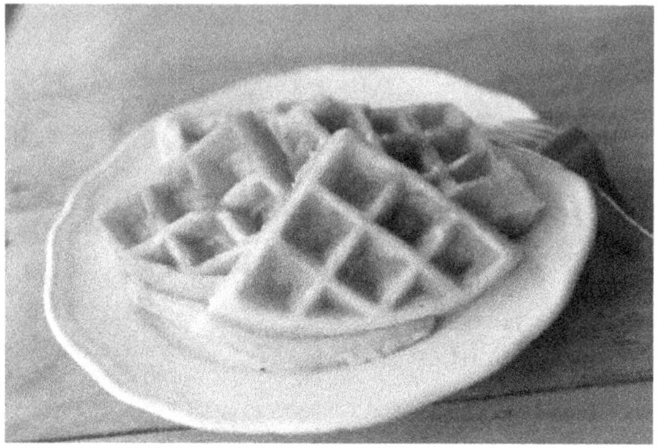

ingredients

Calories: 492

Fat: 32 g

Carbohydrates: 14 g

Protein: 40 g

Cook Time:30 minutes

Servings: 4

- 2 cups cauliflower florets, grated
- ½ tsp garlic powder
- ½ tsp salt
- ½ tsp ground black pepper
- 1 tsp Italian seasoning
- 2 eggs, pasteurized, at room temperature
- 1 cup mozzarella cheese, full-fat, shredded
- 1 cup parmesan cheese, full-fat, shredded

1. Switch on the waffle maker and set it to preheat according to the manufacturer's instructions.
2. Meanwhile, prepare the batter and for this, take a medium-sized bowl, add all the ingredients to it, and whisk well by using an electric mixer at medium speed until incorporated and smooth batter comes together.
3. Grease the waffle maker with avocado oil spray, sprinkle two tablespoons of parmesan cheese on waffle trays until covered, and ladle the prepared batter on top.
4. Shut the waffle maker with its lid and let cook for 5–8 minutes until waffle turns firm and golden-brown.
5. When done, remove waffles by using a tong or a fork and repeat with the remaining batter.
6. Let waffles cool slightly and serve.

Parmesan and Garlic Chaffles

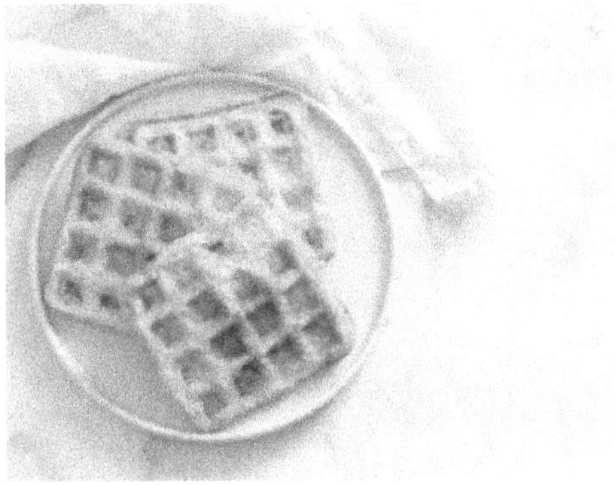

| Ingredients | Calories: 550
Fat: 48 g
Carbohydrates: 8 g
Protein: 54 g | Cook Time:30 minutes
Servings: 4 |

- 1 tsp garlic powder
- 2 cups mozzarella cheese, full-fat, shredded
- 4 eggs, pasteurized, at room temperature
- 1 cup parmesan cheese, full-fat, grated
- 4 teaspoons Italian seasoning

1. Switch on the waffle maker and set it to preheat according to the manufacturer's instructions.
2. Meanwhile, prepare the batter and for this, take a medium-sized bowl, add all the ingredients (except for cheese), whisk until incorporated, and fold in cheese until mixed.
3. Grease the waffle maker with avocado oil spray and ladle the prepared batter on waffle trays.
4. Shut the waffle maker with its lid and let cook for 5–8 minutes until waffle turns firm and golden-brown.
5. When done, remove waffles by using a tong or a fork and repeat with the remaining batter.
6. Let waffles cool slightly and serve.

Pizza Chaffle

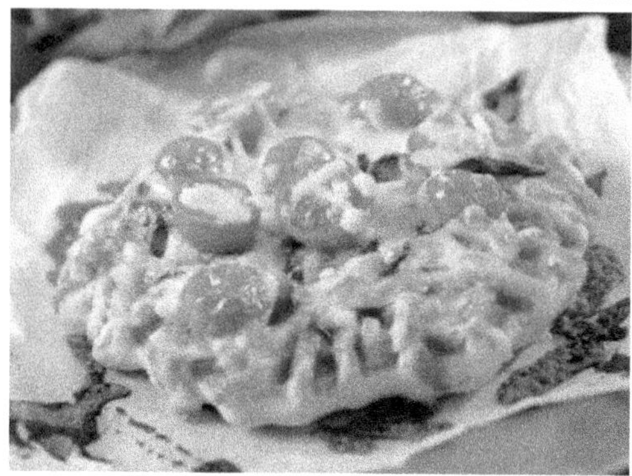

Calories: 530
Fat: 44 g
Carbohydrates: 9 g
Protein: 50 g

Cook Time:30 minutes
Servings: 4

- 4 eggs, pasteurized, at room temperature
- 2 cups mozzarella cheese, full-fat, shredded
- ¼ tsp Italian seasoning
- 4 TBSP pizza sauce, sugar-free
- ½ cup parmesan cheese, grated
- Pepperoni slices, as needed for topping

1. Switch on the waffle maker and set it to preheat according to the manufacturer's instructions.
2. Meanwhile, prepare the batter and for this, take a medium-sized bowl, crack eggs in it, add Italian seasoning and mozzarella cheese, and whisk well by using an electric mixer at medium speed until incorporated and smooth batter comes together.
3. Grease the waffle maker with avocado oil spray, sprinkle 1 tablespoon of parmesan cheese on waffle trays until covered, and ladle the prepared batter on top.
4. Shut the waffle maker with its lid and let cook for 5–8 minutes until waffle turns firm and golden-brown.
5. When done, remove waffles by using a tong or a fork and repeat with the remaining batter.
6. Let waffles cool slightly, spread pizza sauce over each waffle, and top with pepperoni and some more mozzarella cheese.
7. Microwave each waffle for 20 seconds at a high heat setting and then serve.

Buffalo Chicken Chaffle

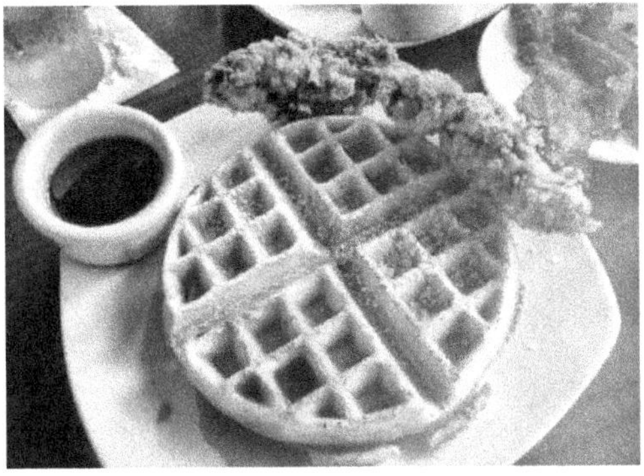

<table>
<tr><td>Ingredients</td><td>Calories: 630
Fat: 48 g
Carbohydrates: 9 g
Protein: 55 g</td><td>Cook Time: 30 minutes
Servings: 4</td></tr>
</table>

- ½ cup celery, diced
- ½ cup almond flour
- 1 cup chicken, pasteurized, shredded
- 2 tsp baking powder
- ½ cup Frank red hot sauce and more for topping
- 4 eggs, pasteurized, at room temperature
- ½ cup mozzarella cheese, full-fat, shredded
- ½ cup feta cheese, full-fat, crumbled
- 1 ½ cup cheddar cheese, full-fat, shredded

1. Take a small bowl, place flour in it, and stir in the baking powder until mixed, set aside until required.
2. Switch on the waffle maker and set it to preheat according to the manufacturer's instructions.
3. Meanwhile, prepare the batter and for this, take a medium-sized bowl, crack eggs in it, and whisk until blended.
4. Beat in red hot sauce, beat in flour mixture until incorporated, beat in all the cheeses until well combined, and then fold in chicken.
5. Grease the waffle maker with avocado oil spray and ladle the prepared batter on waffle trays.
6. Shut the waffle maker with its lid and let cook for 5–8 minutes until waffle turns firm and golden-brown.
7. When done, remove waffles by using a tong or a fork and repeat with the remaining batter.
8. Let waffles cool slightly, top with some more hot sauce and feta cheese, and serve.

Cheddar Chaffles

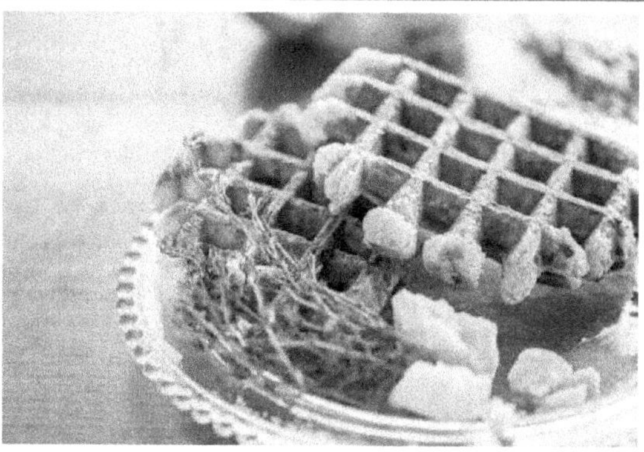

Calories: 550
Fat: 48 g
Carbohydrates: 8 g
Protein: 54 g

Cook Time:30 minutes
Servings: 4

- 4 TBSP almond flour
- 2 cups cheddar cheese, full-fat, shredded
- 4 eggs, pasteurized, at room temperature

1. Switch on the waffle maker and set it to preheat according to the manufacturer's instructions.
2. Meanwhile, prepare the batter and for this, take a medium-sized bowl, add all the ingredients, and whisk well by using an electric mixer at medium speed until incorporated and smooth batter comes together.
3. Grease the waffle maker with avocado oil spray and ladle the prepared batter on waffle trays.
4. Shut the waffle maker with its lid and let cook for 5–8 minutes until waffle turns firm and golden-brown.
5. When done, remove waffles by using a tong or a fork and repeat with the remaining batter.
6. Let waffles cool slightly and serve.

Egg and Mozzarella Chaffle

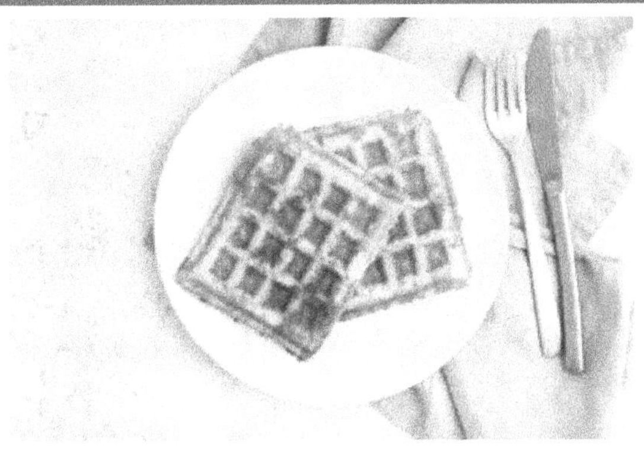

Ingredients		
	Calories: 550	Cook Time:30 minutes
	Fat: 38 g	
	Carbohydrates: 6 g	Servings: 4
	Protein: 35 g	

- 4 eggs, pasteurized, at room temperature
- 2 cups mozzarella cheese, full-fat, shredded

1. Switch on the waffle maker and set it to preheat according to the manufacturer's instructions.
2. Meanwhile, prepare the batter and for this, take a medium-sized bowl, crack eggs in it, add cheese, and whisk well until incorporated and smooth batter comes together.
3. Grease the waffle maker with avocado oil spray and ladle the prepared batter on waffle trays.
4. Shut the waffle maker with its lid and let cook for 5–8 minutes until waffle turns firm and golden-brown.
5. When done, remove waffles by using a tong or a fork and repeat with the remaining batter.
6. Let waffles cool slightly and serve.

Jalapeno and Cheddar Chaffle

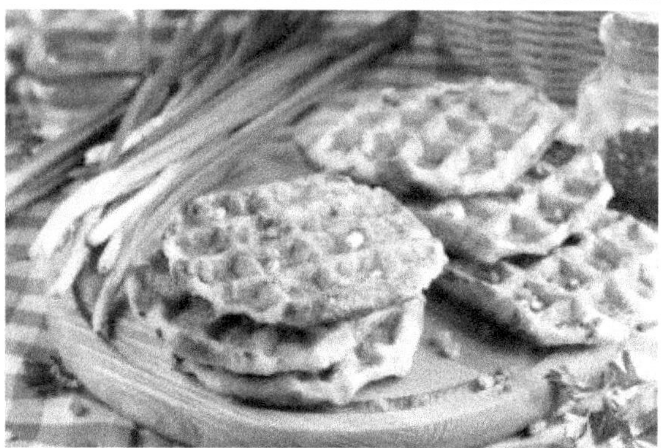

Calories: 560
Fat: 35 g
Carbohydrates: 9 g
Protein: 47 g

Cook Time:30 minutes
Servings: 4

- 4 TBSP jalapenos, chopped
- 4 TBSP almond flour
- 4 eggs, pasteurized, at room temperature
- 2 cups cheddar cheese, full-fat, shredded

1. Switch on the waffle maker and set it to preheat according to the manufacturer's instructions.
2. Meanwhile, prepare the batter and for this, take a medium-sized bowl, crack eggs in it, add remaining ingredients, and whisk well by using an electric mixer at medium speed until incorporated and smooth batter comes together.
3. Grease the waffle maker with avocado oil spray and ladle the prepared batter on waffle trays.
4. Shut the waffle maker with its lid and let cook for 5–8 minutes until waffle turns firm and golden-brown.
5. When done, remove waffles by using a tong or a fork and repeat with the remaining batter.
6. Let waffles cool slightly and serve.

Beef and Onion Bun Chaffle

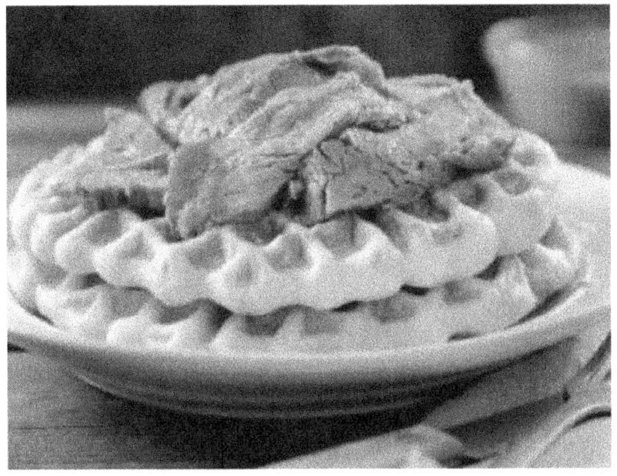

<table>
<tr><td>Ingredients</td><td>Calories: 590
Fat: 40 g
Carbohydrates: 6 g
Protein: 22 g</td><td>Cook Time:30 minutes
Servings: 4</td></tr>
</table>

Sauce	Chaffle
• 8 TBSP horseradish	• 4 TBSP white onion, minced
• 8 tsp erythritol sweetener	• ½ tsp salt
• 1 tsp salt	• 2 cups mozzarella cheese, full-fat, grated
• 2 cups mayonnaise, full-fat	• 4 eggs, pasteurized, at room temperature
	• 16 oz deli roast beef

1. Prepare the sauce and for this, take a medium-sized bowl, place all of its ingredients in it, and whisk until combined. Set aside until needed.
2. Switch on the waffle maker and set it to preheat according to the manufacturer's instructions.
3. Meanwhile, prepare the batter and for this, take a medium-sized bowl, crack eggs in it, add onion, salt, and cheese, and whisk well by using an electric mixer at medium speed until incorporated and smooth batter comes together.
4. Grease the waffle maker with avocado oil spray and ladle the prepared batter on waffle trays.
5. Shut the waffle maker with its lid and let cook for 5–8 minutes until waffle turns firm and golden-brown.
6. When done, remove waffles by using a tong or a fork and repeat with the remaining batter.
7. Let waffles cool slightly, drizzle 2 tablespoons of the horseradish sauce over two waffles, top with beef, and cover the other waffles.
8. Serve chaffle buns with the remaining horseradish sauce, and then serve.

Belgian Chaffles

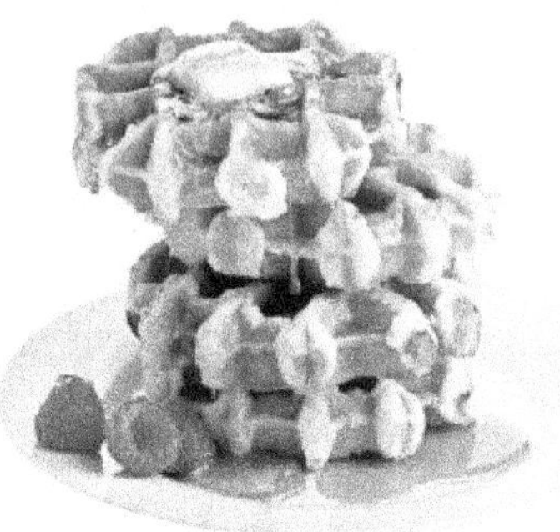

Calories: 480
Fat: 45 g
Carbohydrates: 9 g
Protein: 45 g

Cook Time:30 minutes
Servings: 4

3 cups cheddar and jack cheese blend, full-fat, shredded

4 eggs, pasteurized, at room temperature

1. Switch on the waffle maker and set it to preheat according to the manufacturer's instructions.
2. Meanwhile, prepare the batter and for this, take a medium-sized bowl, crack eggs in it, and whisk until blended.
3. Add cheese blend into the eggs and stir until combined.
4. Grease the waffle maker with avocado oil spray and ladle the prepared batter on waffle trays.
5. Shut the waffle maker with its lid and let cook for 5–8 minutes until waffle turns firm and golden-brown.
6. When done, remove waffles by using a tong or a fork and repeat with the remaining batter.
7. Let waffles cool slightly and serve.

Broccoli and Cheese Chaffle

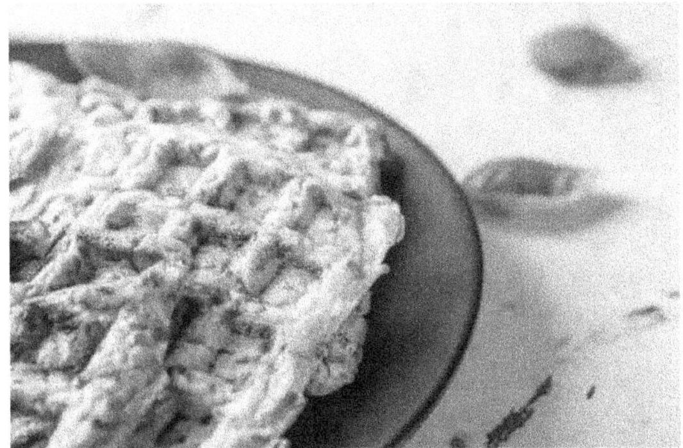

Calories: 460
Fat: 28 g
Carbohydrates: 6 g
Protein: 25 g

Cook Time: 30 minutes
Servings: 4

- 4 TBSP almond flour
- 1 cup broccoli florets, chopped
- 1 tsp garlic powder
- 4 eggs, pasteurized, at room temperature
- 2 cups cheddar cheese, full-fat, shredded

1. Switch on the waffle maker and set it to preheat according to the manufacturer's instructions.
2. Meanwhile, prepare the batter and for this, take a medium-sized bowl, crack eggs in it, add flour, cheese, and garlic powder, and then whisk well by using an electric mixer at medium speed until incorporated and smooth batter comes together.
3. Grease the waffle maker with avocado oil spray, spread half the broccoli into the waffle tray, and ladle the prepared batter on top.
4. Shut the waffle maker with its lid and let cook for 5–8 minutes until waffle turns firm and golden-brown.
5. When done, remove waffles by using a tong or a fork and repeat with the remaining batter and broccoli.
6. Let waffles cool slightly and serve.

Bacon Chaffles

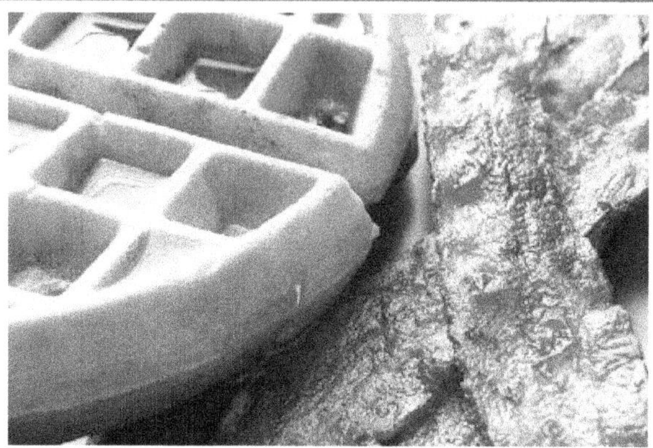

Ingredients

Calories: 590
Fat: 40 g
Carbohydrates: 6 g
Protein: 22 g

Cook Time: 30 minutes
Servings: 4

- 4 TBSP green onion, chopped
- 1 TBSP almond flour
- ½ cup bacon, pasteurized, chopped
- ½ tsp baking powder
- 4 eggs, pasteurized, at room temperature
- 1 cup cheddar cheese, full-fat, shredded
- 1 cup mozzarella cheese, full-fat

1. Switch on the waffle maker and set it to preheat according to the manufacturer's instructions.
2. Meanwhile, prepare the batter and for this, take a medium-sized bowl, crack eggs in it, add flour, baking powder, and both kinds of cheese, and whisk well until incorporated.
3. Add bacon and onion, and stir until mixed and smooth batter comes together.
4. Grease the waffle maker with avocado oil spray and ladle the prepared batter on waffle trays.
5. Shut the waffle maker with its lid and let cook for 5–8 minutes until waffle turns firm and golden-brown.
6. When done, remove waffles by using a tong or a fork and repeat with the remaining batter.
7. Let waffles cool slightly and serve.

Cannabis Chaffles

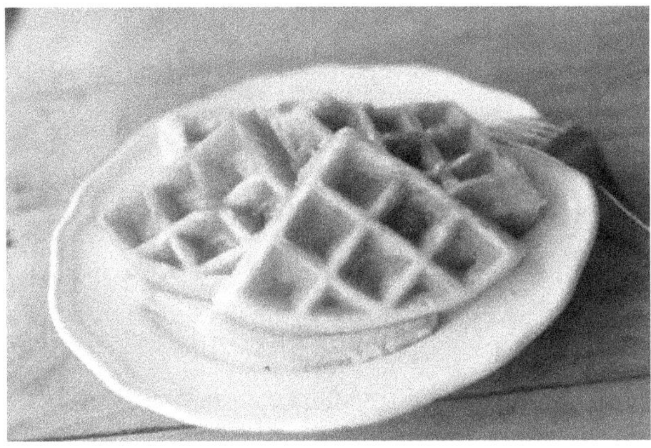

Ingredients

Calories: 422
Fat: 37 g
Carbohydrates: 6 g
Protein: 18 g

Cook Time: 30 minutes
Servings: 4

- 2 tablespoons melted cannabutter
- 1 cup mozzarella cheese, full-fat, shredded
- 1 cup cream cheese, full-fat, softened
- 4 eggs, pasteurized, at room temperature

1. Switch on the waffle maker and set it to preheat according to the manufacturer's instructions.
2. Meanwhile, prepare the batter and for this, take a medium-sized bowl, crack eggs in it, add remaining ingredients, and whisk well by using an electric mixer at medium speed until incorporated and smooth batter comes together.
3. Grease the waffle maker with avocado oil spray and ladle the prepared batter on waffle trays.
4. Shut the waffle maker with its lid and let cook for 5–8 minutes until waffle turns firm and golden-brown.
5. When done, remove waffles by using a tong or a fork and repeat with the remaining batter.
6. Let waffles cool slightly and serve.

Conclusion

We choose a low-carb diet for a variety of reasons. It is needed for those who want to lose weight, athletes, and, first of all, for people with diabetes. Indeed, the consumption of carbohydrates in large quantities is harmful to health and shape since carbohydrates are quickly processed by the body into fats.

All sweet and starchy foods contain carbohydrates. Therefore, a keto diet means giving up chocolates, cookies, and other joys in life. But most of us love sweets. More recently, the diet has become a great stress for the body. Many people are familiar with the situation: being on a diet, you walk past your favorite pastry shop and cannot stand it …

Now, thanks to our book, you can enjoy your favorite recipes without fear for your health and shape!